Inspiring the Inspirational:

Words of Hope from Nurses to Nurses

Sue Heacock, RN, MBA, COHN-S

authorHOUSE®

AuthorHouse™
1663 Liberty Drive, Suite 200
Bloomington, IN 47403
www.authorhouse.com
Phone: 1-800-839-8640

First published by AuthorHouse 10/28/2008

ISBN: 978-1-4389-2233-1 (sc)

Library of Congress Control Number: 2008910130

Printed in the United States of America
Bloomington, Indiana

This book is printed on acid-free paper.

Foreward

I dedicate this book to the professional nurses who selflessly give to those around them every day. To the men and women who share their compassion, hearts, minds, and experience with the less fortunate. To the men and women who don't work simply for a paycheck - but for the payment in kind received from those they touch. Although unable to list them all, I would like to thank the 50+ nursing organizations that agreed to publicize my endeavor and help me discover the great stories you are about to read. Thanks to the nurses around the country (and one in Canada) who submitted stories of love, hope, and compassion that made this work possible. My wish is that this book will truly touch at least one nurse or prospective nurse and serve to remind them of the importance of all they do.

I would like to thank six special people in my life. To my mom and dad for supporting me in any crazy endeavor I ever imagined; for teaching me the importance of hard work; and for always being there (even at the high school basketball games when I was playing the position of "bench warmer"). To George, my 19 year-old Marine, who has taught me anything is possible and no life circumstances should ever limit you from following your dreams. To Jill, my 15 year-old daughter, who has proven that sarcasm is an art form and love conquers all. Thanks to Lynda for years of friendship and her editing skills. Finally, I am indebted to Mark for showing me it is never too late for second chances.

Sue is a Registered Nurse. She resides in Tampa, Florida where she practices as an Occupational Health Nurse. She contributes weekly articles to www.nursetogether.com.

Table Of Contents

NOTE: Names, locations, and details contained in the following stories have been changed to keep the identity of any persons mentioned confidential.

1

Philosophies
To Think About

"If most of us are ashamed of shabby clothes and shoddy furniture, let us be more ashamed of shabby ideas and shoddy philosophies."

~ Albert Einstein

Nursing Is An Art

Nursing is an art;
and if it is to be made an art,
it requires as exclusive a devotion,
as hard a preparation,
as any painter's or sculptor's work;

for what is the having to do with
dead canvas or cold marble,
compared with having to do with the
living body - the temple of God's spirit?

It is one of the Fine Arts;
I had almost said
the finest of the Fine Arts

~ Florence Nightingale

"Caring is the essence of nursing."
~ Jean Watson

"Bound by paperwork, short on hands, sleep, and energy... nurses are rarely short on caring."
~ Sharon Hudacek, *"A Daybook for Nurses"*

"Nurses - one of the few blessings of being ill."
~ Sara Moss-Wolfe

"Service to others is the rent you pay for your room here on earth."
~ Mohammed Ali

"He who has health has hope, and he who has hope has everything."
  ~ Arab Proverb

"Not only must we be good, but we must also be good for something."
  ~ Henry David Thoreau

"During my second year of nursing school our professor gave us a quiz. I breezed through the questions until I read the last one: "What is the first name of the woman who cleans the school?" Surely this was a joke. I had seen the cleaning woman several times, but how would I know her name? I handed in my paper, leaving the last question blank. Before the class ended, one student asked if the last question would count toward our grade. "Absolutely", the professor said. "In your careers, you will meet many people. All are significant. They deserve your attention and care, even if all you do is smile and say hello." I've never forgotten that lesson. I also learned her name was Dorothy."
  ~ Joann C. Jones

"I am only one, but I am one. I cannot do everything, but I can do something. And I will not let what I cannot do interfere with what I can do."
  ~ Edward Everett Hale

Abundant Harvest

Nursing is a very challenging field. Don't let anybody tell you any differently. Nurses will always be needed. We may not always be appreciated or understood, but we bring understanding, nurturing, teaching, and soul searching to others. Most nursing jobs will not bring you financial wealth; however, being a nurse can enrich your life both emotionally and spiritually. We pass these enrichments onto others to make a difference in their lives. We may not always be popular, but we always know the value of a human being. What we know we can teach, and what we teach can spread and grow. That, my friend, yields an abundant harvest!

Jane A. Humphreys, RN. ADN
St Louis, Missouri

"Go the extra mile. It's never crowded."
~ Author Unknown

"We all live under the same sky, but we don't have the same horizon."
~ Konrad Adenauer

An Old Lady's Poem

When an elderly lady died in the geriatric ward of a small hospital near Dundee, in Scotland, it was felt that she had nothing left of any value. Later, when the nurses were going through her meager possessions, they found this poem. Its quality and content so impressed the staff that copies were made and distributed to every nurse in the hospital. One nurse took her copy to Ireland. The old lady's sole bequest to posterity has since appeared in the Christmas edition of the News Magazine of the North Ireland Association for Mental Health. A slide presentation has also been made based on her simple, but eloquent, poem. ... And this little old Scottish lady, with nothing left to give to the world, is now the author of this "anonymous" poem winging across the Internet. Goes to show that we all leave "SOME footprints in time".....

What do you see, nurses, what do you see?
What are you thinking when you're looking at me?
A crabby old woman, not very wise,
Uncertain of habit, with faraway eyes?
Who dribbles her food and makes no reply,
When you say in a loud voice, "I do wish you'd try!"

Who seems not to notice the things that you do,
And forever is missing a stocking or shoe.....
Who, resisting or not, lets you do as you will,
With bathing and feeding, the long day to fill....
Is that what you're thinking? Is that what you see?
Then open your eyes, nurse; you're not looking at me.

I'll tell you who I am as I sit here so still,
As I do at your bidding, as I eat at your will.
I'm a small child of ten ... with a father and mother,
Brothers and sisters, who love one another.

A young girl of sixteen, with wings on her feet,
Dreaming that soon now a lover she'll meet.
A bride soon at twenty -- my heart gives a leap,
Remembering the vows that I promised to keep.
At twenty-five now, I have young of my own,
Who need me to guide and a secure happy home.
A woman of thirty, my young now grown fast,
Bound to each other with ties that should last.
At forty, my young sons have grown and are gone,
But my man's beside me to see I don't mourn.
At fifty once more, babies play round my knee,
Again we know children, my loved one and me.

Dark days are upon me, my husband is dead,
I look at the future, I shudder with dread.
For my young are all rearing young of their own,
And I think of the years and the love that I've known.
I'm now an old woman ... and nature is cruel;
'Tis jest to make old age look like a fool.
The body, it crumbles, grace and vigor depart,
There is now a stone where I once had a heart.
But inside this old carcass a young girl still dwells,
And now and again my battered heart swells.

I remember the joys, I remember the pain,
And I'm loving and living life over again.
I think of the years .... all too few, gone too fast,
And accept the stark fact that nothing can last.

So open your eyes, nurses, open and see,
Not a crabby old woman; look closer ... see ME!!

Remember this poem when you next meet an old person who you might brush aside without looking at the young soul within...... We will one day be there, too!

The above story reproduced with permission from Christy Jones, RN. Found at her website: http://www.nursesareangels.com/nursing_poems.htm

"Growing older isn't upsetting; being perceived as old is."
~ Kenny Rogers

2

Kids And Nursing

"When I approach a child, he inspires me in two sentiments: tenderness for what he is, and respect for what he may become."

~ Louis Pasteur

Rabies

It was my first day as the school nurse many years ago. I was being shown around campus by the headmaster. A first grader came running up and asked the headmaster who I was. She introduced me and the student said, "Thank God. I fell down yesterday and cut my finger. I think I have rabies." He looked at me with bright blue eyes and asked me if I could take the rabies away so he didn't make his dog sick!

Sue Heacock, RN, MBA, COHN-S
Tampa, Florida

Pink Eye Has Spread To My Head

A child came into my office one day to be checked for pink eye. He had a history of seasonal allergies and told me he had "the pink eye" before. It was determined that he was suffering from allergies and he was sent back to class. Later in the day, after running around at recess, he entered his classroom and was scratching his head. He walked up to the teacher and stated, "Now I have the pink head!"

Shawnee Montierth, RN
Meridian, Idaho

"If you can dream it, you can do it."
~ Walt Disney

Rotavirus Or Rabies?

As a school nurse, I have a variety of challenges. One day one of them walked through the door. This spunky third grader was wearing his winter coat, gloves, hat, and had his backpack in hand. He was also wearing a smile from ear to ear. He proudly announced he needed to go home early because he had rotavirus. I wondered about this story, as his mother worked in a local hospital and was very familiar with rotavirus and its degree of contagion.

I asked the young man how many times he had pooped at school that day. "One really big one!" he exclaimed excitedly. I assured him this was normal and he could stay at school. I told him rotavirus is very contagious and if he pooped again I would need to see it. Both appalled and incredulous he exclaimed, "You want to see my pooh!" I assured him that was part of my job. He left and promised to come back if he had to go again.

I found his teacher to explain our conversation. She was very surprised as earlier in the day this same student had told her he had rabies. I told her to keep him in class unless he began foaming at the mouth.

What a busy day for this young man!

Heather Meador, RN, BSN
Solon, Iowa

"Children are likely to live up to what you believe of them."
~ Lady Bird Johnson

Suddenly Stricken

I am not your typical school nurse. I am male, six feet-two inches tall, and weigh 200 pounds. Frequently, parents, school visitors, and new teachers mistake me for a campus security officer or an administrator.

One day several years ago, I looked up to see a small girl walking down the hall toward the health office. What was unusual was that she had her head tipped back, eyes closed; and was erratically waving both extended arms in front of her. She was accompanied by two other girls from her class.

What was the reason for the second grader's visit to the health office? She had been suddenly stricken blind when the teacher handed out an arithmetic test. Her two companions were all atwitter in their concern, right up until the "blind" girl's eyes popped wide open and she blurted out, "You can't be the nurse, you're a BOY!"

JT Hayes, RN, PHN
Palm Springs, California

JT's email quote:
"Men fight for liberty and win it with hard knocks.
Their children, brought up easy, let it slip away again, poor fools.
And their grand-children are once more slaves."
~ D. H. Lawrence (1885-1938)

Least Favorite Subject In School

A louse is a louse, is a louse, is a louse,
Especially on your head or in your house.
No worse when it rides into our schools,
But head lice are against the rules.

It's just a bug, no relation to dirt,
Causes itching, but does not hurt.
But embarrassing it is for sure,
Luckily there's a simple cure.

Lice shampoo for every head,
Clean clothes, furniture, brush, and bed.
And hope nevermore to see bugs roam,
Not in school and not in your home.

If your child begins some scratching,
Check to see if something is hatching.
The louse's goal is just to survive,
For your comfort, lice must not stay alive.

Roberta Moore, RN, PHN
Shafter, California

"A child is not a vase to be filled, but a fire to be lit."
~ Rabelais

Charlie And Daniel

On his first day of school his mother dropped him off and drove away. No one knew who he was or where he belonged. We speculated, by his size, that he belonged in kindergarten. He refused to talk to anyone and so his teacher named him Charlie. When she called his name he had no facial expression nor did he turn to look at her. After a few days the teacher managed to make contact with his mother who was parked in the school parking lot near the end of the day. She found out Charlie's real name, address, and all the other information required for school admission. Charlie took medication on a daily basis and would come into my office each day to take his pill before lunch. He never said a word.

I had been asked by a friend at church if I would be willing to make puppets for the newly formed puppet troop; as I have a little known sewing talent! Of course I said I would try so I went to a class on puppet making and made my first puppet. I named him Daniel. Daniel was a brown skinned, dark eyed, bald headed Muppet-like puppet who sported a blue blazer. I brought him to my office and sat him on the corner of my desk so I could display my latest accomplishment. I never dreamt the impact Daniel would make on the children at my school.

Charlie came in the office the first day Daniel was there and immediately asked, "Who's that?" I was so shocked that Charlie was talking that I could hardly talk myself. I told him, "His name is Daniel and he is a very good friend of mine." Charlie said, "Oh" then took his medication and left my office without another word. Charlie repeated this same routine for several days until one day he asked permission to speak with Daniel. I told him that Daniel is always willing to listen to him anytime.

The teacher and I conferred and decided that Charlie could come to my office any afternoon at a set time and talk with Daniel. Charlie came everyday at 2:15 and would spend 15 minutes talking with Daniel. Daniel just sat on the corner of my desk and listened. I would keep myself busy in my office but listen to what Charlie was saying to Daniel. Charlie told Daniel the details of his life; from his mom prostituting, to his mom selling drugs, to no food in the house, to hiding in the closet when his mom was angry, to running away when the police came to the door, to being thrown out of a second story window. He went on and on.

One afternoon Charlie stopped by to say goodbye to Daniel. He said he was moving out of state the next day. He asked it if would be okay with me if he gave Daniel something. Of course I said yes. Charlie dug into his pocket and pulled out a small halo pin that he had received from the church across the street for being at breakfast each morning. I helped Charlie pin the halo onto Daniel's lapel. Charlie shook his head and said to Daniel, "You are the best friend I have ever had." He turned around and walked out. I never saw Charlie again, but each time I see Daniel and his halo pin, I say a little prayer for Charlie.

Anna M. Hines, RN, MPH
Altoona, Iowa

"If you can't hold children in your arms, please hold them in your heart."
~ Mother Clara Hale

"I'm Dying"

Motherhood and school nursing have a common thread....you are never really prepared. That first year as an elementary school nurse I was trying to be very professional during each interaction with students and used my best interviewing and assessment skills. Not that I don't still do a good job, but after 14 years on the job, I can sniff out a "faker" by the rhythmic exaggerated limp; mounting moans if I don't say the magic works, "looks like you will have to go home", and the student's eagerness to furnish the phone numbers of extended family members in three states.

Eight-year old Howie was a picture. He stood out in any classroom. He was the kid whose name and face you remember from the first second you meet. Early on a beautiful fall day, Howie presented himself in the doorway of my tiny office with tube socks pulled up tight, shorts a size too small, a polo shirt, tousled dark curly hair badly in need of a cut, and taped up glasses. All he lacked was the pocket protector. If Charles Schultz had ever met Howie, I am confident he would have made Howie a PEANUTS character.

Howie proceeded to very matter-of-factly inform me that he needed to go home and I should call his mom right away. I explained that I couldn't automatically call home without first taking his temperature and checking him out. When Howie displayed no temperature or any confirmable symptoms, his list of aches and pains started to multiply. Further questioning and examination revealed no real malady. Howie was obviously dismayed that a "go home" commitment from his strict rookie school nurse was still nowhere in sight.

Sensing a losing hand, Howie went for his ace in the hole. "Actually Ms. Wetenkamp, I'm dying." Startled and intrigued by his statement, all I could think to say was, "Gosh Howie, I've never died before. Tell me what it's like." His oh-so serious reply was, "Well, it's a lot like diarrhea."

Through tears disguised as "something in my eye" I dialed Howie's mother. She explained that Howie's grandmother was flying in from Georgia and Howie's sudden case of the deadly runs was probably just a ploy to get out of school on this special occasion. Of course I let him go – I'm a tough nurse, but a marshmallow soft grandma!

Becky Wetenkamp, RN, BSN
Plattsmouth, NE

"Every adult needs a child to teach; it's the way adults learn."
~ Frank A. Clark

Growing With My Patient
The Story of a Pediatric Office Nurse

A call from the nursery: "Let me talk to the nurse."
"Dr. Krohn has a baby at Methodist. Baby Boy Schmitz."

Two days old, newborn call: baby not sleeping.

Five days old, Mom calls: fussy baby. Reassure. Listen. Educate.

Seven days old. Dad calls: baby spitting up. Listen. Reassure. Educate.

Two weeks old. Mom calls: still no sleep, still spitting up.
Coming in for check up in morning.

Two months old. Formula changed. Still spitting up.
Listen. Reassure. Educate.

Six weeks old. Mom calls: baby acne.
Reassure. Educate.

Four months old. Diarrhea.
Listen. Reassure. Educate.

Six months old. Feeding solids.
Reassure. Educate. Follow-up.

Nine months old. Flying to Grandma's. What to do in the plane?
Discuss comforting measures. "Have a good trip."

Eighteen months old. Had immunizations. Lump at injection site. Reassure. Educate.

Two and a half years old. Mom pregnant. "I remember all the good advice from before.
What about sibling rivalry?"
Congratulate. Reassure. Listen. Educate.

Three years old. "Haven't seen you in awhile."

Four years old. "My, how he's grown!"

Five years old. "Kindergarten already?"

Junior high. So busy.
Encourage healthy behaviors. Laugh. Enjoy.

College.
"Have I really known you all these years?"
"Seems like only yesterday…"
"Where are you going to school?"

A call from the nursery: "Let me talk to the nurse."
"Dr. Krohn has a baby at Methodist.
Baby Girl Schmitz."
I know her dad!

Sue Grady Bristol, RN, BSN
Omaha, Nebraska

"We can do no great things, only small things with great love."
~ Mother Teresa

The Pledge Of Allegiance

It was my first day as a school nurse in a multi-handicapped classroom. Upon entering the room, my eyes fell upon a little boy in a wheelchair; his seemingly lifeless left arm lying close to his body. I found out his name was Timothy and he had a twin brother in another classroom who had no handicaps. Timothy had cerebral palsy and difficulty speaking. He refused to talk. As I met and partnered with his physical and occupational therapists, it was felt that Timothy had the potential to talk and walk with assistance but didn't seem motivated to try.

My first step was to develop a trusting relationship with Timothy. I would spend time just holding him as I read or sang to him. I was actively involved in his therapy and asked to assist in feeding him. There would be times I would take him out of the classroom alone and spend special time with him. In such instances we would go to the library or I would wheel him outside to look at the flowers or birds.

My first success was the day I brought in a Beach Boys cassette and discovered Timothy's love for music. There was a particular song that made his eyes light up and brought a smile to his face. I was determined to get him to recognize his unused left arm. It was as if we had to teach his brain to re-recognize the arm as a part of his body. So when I picked him up I started having him reach up to me with his left arm. His right arm would be wrapped around my neck and I would extend his left arm and we would dance to the Beach Boys song. He would laugh out loud with glee. That was when progress accelerated.

We actively worked on speech lessons. If Timothy would communicate his needs to us, we would then reward him. Each morning we listened to the Pledge of Allegiance and over time Timothy would attempt to say some of the words. A goal was set that by the end of next year we would have Timothy independently recite the entire Pledge of Allegiance over the school intercom.

As his speech improved so did his mobility. Little by little his legs became stronger with physical therapy and he started using a walker. His reward would be to walk to the principal's office (this was a positive thing). He was excelling by leaps and bounds!

The next school year I found out I was going to be moving out of the area. It broke my heart. As a farewell gift to me, my coworkers and Timothy worked even harder on the Pledge of Allegiance. My last week at the school Timothy recited the Pledge of Allegiance over the school intercom during morning announcements. I listened with tears rolling down my cheeks and could never have imagined receiving a better gift.

It was seven years later I received a phone call from a former coworker. She informed me that Timothy had died. After shedding tears of sadness, I sat down and wrote Timothy's mother about the many happy memories I had of Timothy. She wrote me a thank you note and shared how much she appreciated all I had done for Timothy. We were both comforted.

I started out wanting to make a positive change in Timothy's life. I ended up learning that in every child, no matter their "disability" or "handicap" love, trust, and encouragement can make miracles happen.

Brenda Lindahl, RN, School Nurse
Loachapoka, Alabama

Harold The Bear

About a year ago a boy of twelve moved into our hospital's coverage area. This young man had Cystic Fibrosis and was frequently in our Emergency Department (ED). He was usually very ill and both he and his mother scared when he came for treatment. It is an "unwritten policy" that whoever triages a patient keeps him/her throughout the ED stay. In November 2007, it became my turn to care for the little boy.

When he arrived he was very short of breath, with O2 sats in the mid 80s and a pulse in the 130s. He looked extremely sick. I took him straight to a room and began to reassure him and his mother as I got my equipment and supplies and got to work. As I got ready to start his IV and draw labs, he started to cry and said, "Nobody is able to get it on the first try." I patted his shoulder and told him (trying to reassure him) that, "I never try, I get it done" (all the while praying to myself). He smiled and promised he would hold still for me…SUCCESS….on the first stick I got a good solid line, drew labs, and got his medications on board. Both he and his mom hugged me and thanked me for getting it the first time. A few hours later he was much improved and left without an admission. Here comes the kicker……….

Every time he subsequently came to the ED he would ask for me to take care of him! My co-workers were more than happy to oblige. I was always cheerful and did my best with him. I never missed an IV or blood draw on him. I attribute this to 25 years as a Paramedic and the many prayers I said during each IV start! One day his mother came to the ED with a sibling and told me that my favorite patient was not doing well, however, he had sent a message for me.

Seems he went to a "Build-a-Bear" store and built a large teddy bear and dressed it in scrubs. He told his mom that since I couldn't follow him to the tertiary hospital that "Harold the Nurse-Bear" would have to.

The young man and his family have since moved out of state to be closer to a larger facility and more specialized care. I will never forget him and whenever I get discouraged I think of a small, skinny boy holding a teddy bear named after me.

Harold Ellison, RN
Soldotna, Alaska

"Nurses dispense comfort, compassion, and caring without even a prescription."

~ Val Saintsbury

3

Nurses Inspiring Nurses

"Inspiration is never genuine if it is known as inspiration at the time. True inspiration always steals on a person, its importance not being fully recognized for some time."

~ Samuel Butler

Still Nursing At 90

The following article was written for publication in a local newspaper. The author agreed to share it with us. I have also included suggestions to be still nursing at 90 from nurses around the globe. Enjoy!

The other night, my husband and I were watching television when someone on a commercial stated something about retiring at age 90. I didn't hear the rest of the dialogue because I was rolling on the floor and laughing too hard at the visual images I was getting of my own future. As a baby boomer that is not independently wealthy, I fully expect that the words, "I'm retired" will not be coming from my lips in this lifetime.

I have written in my newspaper column that I often wonder what my future will be. I love hospice nursing and feel a deep pull towards the sacred work I do everyday. The advantage I have now is that I'm relatively healthy and feel motivated and excited about my daily work. So, as I gaze into my crystal ball to see what the future brings, this is what I see.

Here's my ideal work day at age 90. I wake up each morning without an alarm clock. I don't feel rushed, as my employer has assured me that my sleep is important so that my work day doesn't include a lot of errors. I take my time getting ready and my hired cook has my breakfast ready for me, warm on the table. I leisurely enjoy my food and steaming cup of Joe with my sweetie (husband) who will be 92 when I'm 90. We do so love to be together!

My limousine driver knocks on the front door and announces that it's time to get my day started. It's now about 10:30 AM. I casually collect my notebook, nursing bag, and laptop computer (can't do without it!) and he slowly escorts me and my walker to the curb. He kindly assists me into the limo and then my walker is placed in the storage area in the back. I give him the address of my first patient and off we go.

In between patient visits, I enjoy the peace of being inside the limo, with the windows all blacked out and my satellite radio emitting waves of beautiful music. I also like listening to my favorite talk radio hostess, Oprah. She's about 80 now, you know, and still going strong. I especially love it when she features Dr. Oz (age 75 and doing radio shows just for the fun of it, since he's independently wealthy) and Wayne Dyer (also my age and quite rich). They remind the baby boomers how we can improve our lives and live longer by eating right and thinking good thoughts.

As I reach each patient's home, my limo driver helps me out with my walker, and he carries my notebook and laptop computer. Just think! I no longer have to carry these heavy items, and my employer (yep, the compassionate one!) urges me to take care not to lift them so my shoulders can heal from the multiple surgeries I've had to keep the joints moving. My employer had mentioned the term "wheelchair" to me several times, encouraging me to consider using one because he wants my knees to heal properly from my recent joint replacement. I really do not want to consider a wheelchair; because I'm pretty sure that will end my career as a hospice nurse (Did you know that most homes in our town are NOT wheelchair accessible?).

So, that's the way I see it going for me. All these ideas raced through my mind the other night as I contemplated what it would be like to still be working at age 90. All the retirement money I've worked hard to save – will I have time to spend it? I think not, as I'll be out seeing my patients, many of whom will be 20 or 30 years my junior! Keep your eyes peeled for my limo, with the magnetic signed plastered to the side, "Still Nursing at 90!"

Paula Schneider, RN, CHPN, MPH
Minden, Nevada

A little bit about Paula: "My life's mission is to 'lead and inspire myself and others to personal and spiritual health', and this mission is currently best exemplified through my hospice work with those living the last chapter of their lives. In my spare time, I write weekly articles on hospice, death and dying, spirituality, and care giving for Carson City's daily newspaper. In 1997, I published a book of true and inspiring stories written by nurses from all over the world, Healing Hearts. In 2007 I compiled my articles from the newspaper into a compendium of useful training articles for those interested in hospice work."

Paula's tip for still being able to nurse at 90:

"Get plenty of sleep at night, try to eat your fruits and veggies, and surround yourself with loving, positive, and supportive friends."

More Ideas To Still Be Nursing At 90:

"Have one or more meaningful hobbies outside of nursing to maintain an emotional balance and hopefully some objectivity regarding your job."

    Cary Jo Cook, BSN, RN, CMSRN

    Bartlett, Illinois

"Continue to pursue educational opportunities - be they achievement of a PhD (in several areas if you so desire) or take community classes helping you to learn to garden well, write poetry, paint, cook, or whatever."

    Cindi Leigh Wigston, RN CIC

    Orillia, Ontario Canada

"Embrace "new" trends and ideas. Try to avoid being stuck in a time period with clothing, music, and yes even TV shows. Explore the creative talents of the young and up-and-comers. You will feel younger and your mind will be constantly challenged trying to "upgrade".

    Lia M. Anderson APRN, BC

    Alexandria, Virginia

"I think we must also keep in mind to enjoy and appreciate the simple things because even at age 22 I have to take a step back and embrace the ground beneath my feet, the sun on my back, or even the rain on my face. Not every enjoyment must be sought after and financially supported like Yoga classes... just look all around you. I always wake up asking myself, "How can I make this day the best day of my life?" I would also celebrate the fact that I'm 90 years old and still going strong in this messed up world :)"

Rebekah C. Swanson, Nursing Student
Nisswa, Minnesota

"As we grow old, the beauty steals inward."

~ Ralph Waldo Emerson

"If you take too long in deciding what to do with your life, you'll find you've done it."

~ Pam Shaw

The Power Of Education And Experience

I have been a nurse for 21 years and feel there is wisdom with age. My main motivation for becoming a nurse was to be an advocate for people that could not represent themselves in abuse and neglect situations. This includes children, the elderly, and the disabled. I believe this is a common impetus for nurses. Nurses are liaisons. We see patients up close. I have assisted many people recovering from trauma and have made efforts to protect them. That's the bottom line of nursing: saving lives and comforting others.

Education and information can save your life. One prime function in nursing is educating others to maintain health and wellness. I think back to many situations, both on and off the clock, where someone could have died if I hadn't known the right course of action. I even survived some pretty rough situations that very well could have killed me. I remember being homeless due to a longstanding injury from an auto accident. Knowing about the social services system and other support systems helped save me from ending up on the street. Being an educated nurse gave me the knowledge of where to go for help and the ability to remain persistent. Some people don't know those things and get lost in the system. I use what I learned to help others to heal and recover.

I have been on this earth for almost a half of a century. I know I'm not *that* old, or so people older than me tell me.........but I have seen a lot. When I was growing up children did not have human rights. The laws in most states in America were vague and lenient; allowing parents to treat their children as property – like livestock. Child abuse, to include sexual abuse, was a fact of life for many children. Most people lacked training and understanding of child psychology. Many schools did not have a nurse to assist in protecting children and educating the public.

Today child abuse is considered a serious crime. Nurses intervene in child abuse issues a great deal - especially in jobs focusing on children. That's what I do. I am a school nurse in the St. Louis Public School System. We have in-service classes each year about child abuse detection, prevention, and other child protection issues. The quality of life for children has improved because of this education and information. Today's children will be running society some day. Although there is a concern about too much permissiveness for children and not enough teaching of self discipline, I still believe that life for a child is better than when I was young. Part of that can be credited to nurses and our contribution to children.

Nurses are also educated in spiritual issues and psychology for all age groups. We are required to study many different cultures, religions, and philosophies as they apply to mind, body, and spirit. We learn different dietary needs and cultural rituals. When we study psychology, we also learn communication skills that assist us in calming people in stressful and volatile situations. We have more power than we realize.

Jane Humphreys RN, ADN
Saint Louis, Missouri

"Information's pretty thin stuff unless mixed with experience."
~ Clarence Day – *The Crow's Nest*

Jan

When I was fourteen and yet undecided what I would be when I grew up, I developed a ruptured appendix. The nurse who cared for me during my two lengthy hospitalizations left such an impression on me that I decided I would follow in her footsteps. From the moment I met her, I wanted only to be a nurse like "Jan".

About 25 years later, I received a letter from my mother that included a newspaper clipping about Jan and her husband. They were celebrating their 25th wedding anniversary. I had not spoken to Jan during those 25 years, but decided this would be an opportunity for me to tell her how she had changed my life and let her know that I was actively engaged in my own nursing career.

Several weeks later I received a hand-written letter from Jan. She wanted me know that, although she didn't remember me specifically, she was so grateful that I had taken the time to share my thoughts with her. She had recently been diagnosed with Amyotrophic Lateral Sclerosis (ALS) (often referred to as "Lou Gehrig's Disease"). She and her husband were in agreement that as the disease progressed, they would not seek heroic measures to prolong her life. She had already progressed to a point where she was unable to continue caring for patients. She was very sad to be unable to practice the career she loved, but now felt some reassurance that another nurse would be carrying on her love for the profession.

This past year I received another letter from my mother with the clipping of Jan's obituary. Whenever I think of her I recall how the kindness of one dedicated nurse changed my life. It also reminds me that I need to approach each patient with the realization that I may not know what I could be bringing to them as a side effect of my nursing care!

Marti Potter, RN, BSN, MPH
Steamboat Springs, Colorado

"My father always told me to find a job you love and you'll never have to work a day in your life."

~ Jim Fox

It Starts With One

I was so thrilled to be on the "Internet" in 1996, but didn't know where to go and what to look up. I "met" another nurse – Marlene-in a game room and we started to talk. I decided if there were any other nurses on the internet we ought to form a group and support one another. So, Marlene and I started a group with two other nurses. Marlene wrote the newsletter originally - - - a chatty type. I started searching for nurses and our group grew. I named our group Paradigm97 and wrote a mission statement. I now write and post the monthly newsletter. It is dedicated to evidence based nursing, nursing research, medical news, and medical recalls. We are now international and have 450 members.

Frances J. Jessup, RN, BSN
Valdosta, Georgia

What Frances wrote that also inspired me, *"I received my Bachelors in 1995 at the age of 59."*

"If opportunity doesn't knock, build a door."
 ⁓ Milton Berle

Nurse 24-7-365

My journey in nursing has been long, but rewarding. I started as a Certified Nursing Assistant and then became a Licensed Practical Nurse. I still could not get enough of nursing so went back to school and earned my current title of Registered Nurse, BSN. Nursing is an extremely rewarding job and something that I have enjoyed learning more about with each passing day.

One day in 2006 I was making my routine drive to work (if you call an hour and thirty minutes each way routine) when I happened upon a bad vehicle accident. I *naturally stopped* to help, as would all you nurses reading this!

A large concrete mixer vehicle had struck a bridge abutment and the vehicle had massive amounts of damage. I instinctively climbed onto the hood of the truck and assessed and monitored the trapped driver until he was removed from the vehicle. I reassured him right up to the time the helicopter airlifted him to the hospital. Naturally, I felt that I had done my civic duty and wondered how this man was doing over the next few days.

I was both surprised and honored to receive a letter from the employer of the vehicle. The following are excerpt from the letter:

"How fortunate for him that the first person on the scene to render assistance was an RN! The driver has now been released from the hospital, but has a long recovery period ahead of him."

"I'm sure your prompt, careful and professional attention greatly contributed to his quick release from the hospital. It is gratifying to know that there are still individuals who are willing to put their busy schedule on hold and come to the aid of others."

"As a small token of our appreciation for your assistance, please accept this shirt with our company logo. We hope that your wearing it will give you a repeated reminder of your concern for others."

Even if you only hear a special "Thank You" from a handful of people over the years - - that is all you need to keep you inspired.

Jackie Brinkley, RN, BSN
Mount Airy, North Carolina

"A pat on the back, though only a few vertebrae removed from a kick in the pants, is miles ahead in results."

~ Bennett Cerf

Hands Free Restraints

One day while serving as the manager of a medical-surgical unit I received a call from a prospective employer for one of my former nurses. The facility I worked at was a small 40-bed hospital in a rural community. After I gave my former nurse a glowing recommendation, the prospective employer inquired, "My soon to be employee mentioned you have invented a hands-free restraint system. Could you tell me about it?"

I laughed heartily and proceeded to explain my system. I told her, "Our facility can not afford any of the alarm beds on the market to alert us when confused patients are getting out of bed, so we went to the recycle bin. Taking empty soda cans we wash them, flatten them, and place them around the foot of the bed on top of the covers. When a patient begins to stir and throw off his/her lines, the soda cans fall to the tile floor alerting us that the patient is on the move." I continued, "If the patient is stable on his/her feet, but we don't want the patient wandering, we line the floor across the threshold of the room door with empty, non-flattened cans. As the patient shuffles through the door, he/she will literally 'kick the cans' and we know the patient was up and about."

We both laughed. The medical industry has devised all type of bed alert systems; some in the structure of the bed and some add on types. These are all to keep the patient safe without restraining them against their will. Here in our rural community the solution was found in the recycle bin!

Pamela F. Rodkey, RN
Medford, Oregon

"An idea can turn to dust or magic, depending on the talent that rubs against it."

~ William Bernbach

The Good Ole' Days

How often do we hear nursing colleagues wistfully recall their earlier nursing careers?

My first nursing position, following graduation in 1965, was at a large university teaching hospital. I was assigned to a contagious isolation unit where all of the patients suffered from major wound infections.

At that hospital Texas Catheters (external catheters) were unavailable so we were compelled to make them from condoms and rubber tubing. While this task was not overly challenging, the condoms were stored in the locked narcotics cabinet so at the change of each shift we had to count them along with the narcotics. Whichever administrator dreamed this one up apparently thought we were planning to use the condoms for recreational, rather than medical purposes!

Another less than appetizing procedure prevalent at that time was preparation of fecal enemas. Because the patients on our unit were on massive doses of antibiotics the bacterial flora in their colons often was depleted. All of the nurses in the unit dreaded finding a posted notice directing staff to provide fresh stool for the procedure and silently crossed their fingers that no one would fulfill the request on their shift. Usually some eager medical student would oblige and provide his/her "gift to science" to one of us.

We always hoped the donor was not constipated as our task was to mix the stool with saline while macerating it with a wooden tongue blade. Although we were often tempted, especially with cantankerous patients, we resisted the temptation to announce the contents of their dose.

When I sometimes relate these, and other, experiences of the sixties and seventies to today's crop of nurses they suspiciously accuse me of putting them on. But these experiences were quite common practices of that era.

Sandra K. Sharp, MSN, ARNP
Miami Beach, Florida

"We are tomorrow's past."
~ Mary Webb – *Precious Bane*

Aunt Tommy

My father's only sister, my Aunt Tommy (Lillian Beck Fuller) graduated from Presbyterian Hospital School of Nursing in the 1920s and immediately joined the Chicago Visiting Nurse Service (VNS). Her first assignment was the VNS station at Hull House. I grew up hearing her stories of having lunch with Jane Addams, caring for Al Capone's mother, and dodging into doorways to avoid flying bullets.

When Aunt Tommy became a single parent of an 18-month old and a 3-year old during the Great Depression, she returned to her parents' home in Mountain Iron, Minnesota. She was hired by the Works Progress Administration (WPA) to do public health surveys and was the only one in her household employed. When the Mountain Iron school nurse left, Aunt Tommy took over. She was a school nurse in the true public health model of Lillian Wald and Lina Rogers of New York's Henry Street Settlement. She visited homes after school to check on children who had not been at school, conducted well baby and prenatal clinics, and cared for the entire community. For two summers, she took public health courses at the University of Minnesota.

Once her children were grown, she became the nurse at the Minneapolis YMCA's Camp Warren in Eveleth, Minnesota. Garrison Keillor, of Prairie Home Companion fame, was one of the camp counselors and wrote a story about Aunt Tommy for the YMCA magazine.

Aunt Tommy lived into her 90s and was still taking care of her community at the senior housing center that became her last home.

Like Aunt Tommy, I am inspired to excellence by my patients, my students, and my nursing colleagues in all disciplines. I am privileged to practice in an interdisciplinary community health center and to work with an interdisciplinary team to address violence in an old New England mill city. Everyday I feel privileged to be a nurse.

Joellen W. Hawkins, RN, WHNP-BC, PhD
Auburndale, Massachusetts

"Goodness is the only investment that never fails."
~ Henry David Thoreau

Falls Lead To Success

I was raised in the country and when I started first grade was first exposed to the hard black tarry macadam. The school nurse and secretary shared the duties of caring for the children in the elementary school. The secretary alone saw me over 30 times in nine months! I was not known as Miss Graceful! Exasperated one day when I had fallen and scraped my knee twice in the same day she said, "You need to learn to do this yourself." It was said with a smile, but even as a young child, I knew I was pushing the outer limits of her patience.

Twenty-three years later when I was graduating as an LPN, I remembered her words. Thank you, Ms. Zuber for planting the first seeds of nursing in my brain in first grade.

Jeanette Smith, RN, BS
Harrisburg, Pennsylvania

"Be an opener of doors for such as come after thee, and do not try to make the universe a blind alley."
~ Ralph Waldo Emerson

Fate

I was born in the Philippines and hail from a family of thirty Registered Nurses. It all started with my Aunt Phoebe who became an RN in the 1960s. She was followed by her younger sister and then my Aunt Precy. She became the first one in the family to travel to and work in the United States. That is where it all began: cousins and nieces followed in the legacy that Aunt Phoebe had established. Nursing is in the hearts of the younger generation and the number of nurses in my clan continues to grow.

I chose a different path. It was early 1980 when I came to the United States on a scholarship from Brigham Young University in Hawaii. My major was Hotel, Restaurant, and Travel Management. I never realized that I would end up in nursing. But fate had its hand. I was living in a small town in Hawaii and it became apparent that there was a crisis due to the nursing shortage and the demand for nurses everywhere was high.

Upon relocating from Hawaii to California, I started working as a Certified Nursing Assistant (CNA). I worked in a long term care facility helping the elderly. My experiences as a CNA motivated me to consider advancing my education in nursing. So along I went. I was working, going to nursing school, dealing with pregnancy, and raising children. It was not easy. With hard work and strong self-determination, I earned the title of Licensed Vocational Nurse (LVN) in 1990. I worked in an acute care hospital in our area and gained excellent nursing experience as an LVN. Unfortunately, I was not considered a nurse by the doctors I worked with on the floor. Doctors would come into the unit looking for "the nurse" and would ignore me —even if I were standing right in front of them. They meant they wanted to see the Registered Nurse. I endured this treatment and turned it into a challenge to myself to go back to school to become an RN.

I worked my way through RN school working full-time (12-hour night shifts) and still maintaining my wife and mother duties! I struggled every day to manage work, school, and family. When I graduated in 1994 and subsequently passed the state boards, the struggle was fully worth the benefits. Achieving the RN license meant so much to me. Not only did it advance my salary, but it gained me professional respect. I became one of the "nurses" the doctors referred to. It made me feel good to be included in the team and finally be called "The Nurse".

Verna Faune-Wall, RN, BSN, PHN
Visalia, California

"My life is my message."
~ Mahatma Ghandi

4

Simply Funny

"Happy is the person who can laugh at himself.
He will never cease to be amused."

~ Habib Bourguiba

"After two days in the hospital,
I took a turn for the nurse."

~ W.C. Fields

Where Are You Putting That Needle?

An 18-year old female patient brought her mother with her for the patient's first Gardasil vaccine. Her mother and I thought it was because she was nervous about receiving the shot. We soon found out she was nervous because she thought the shot went "down there"! After all, it is a cervical cancer prevention measure. Her mother laughed when the doctor allayed the fear and we assured her the shot would go in her arm or leg just like any other vaccine.

Patricia Stark, RN, MSN, BC, ANP
Waco, Texas

Why Is My Urine Orange?

I saw a 38-year old healthy male patient for treatment of an irritated bug bite on his leg. He was prescribed doxycycline and instructed to take the medication twice a day for 10 days. He called the office after his second dose very concerned because his urine had turned orange! After checking the Physician Desk Reference (PDR) and confirming that this was not a side effect of doxycycline, I called the patient back. He apologized for the confusion and advised me that he had checked with his wife and instead of taking his daily multivitamin, he had taken her Pyridium tablet!

Joe A. Gorelick, NP
Campbell, California

"To err is human; to refrain from laughing, humane."
~ Lane Olinghouse

Payback

Nursing can be fun and full of surprises. When I was in college, we had a sociology term paper assignment on "deviant behaviors". I was working as a student nurse on an all male floor. All patients were in traction of some sort: bucks, striker frames, etc. They decided to play a joke on me at Christmas-time. The wife of one of the patient's brought in eggnog to share with the ward members. It was in a milk carton and I had never tried eggnog before. I took a long sip and began to cough… a lot. The eggnog had been spiked with rum. I was not expecting it and I got a lot of laughs from the patient and his wife.

I have never been accused of letting sleeping dogs lie and decided to get even. When the patient asked me to empty his metal urinal, I went down the hall and did just that. Then I filled it up with ice. The next time the patient used the urinal I heard the echo of "NURSE!" I chuckled for I knew that I had "cooled him down". I only got a "B" on the assignment because I had failed to consider the sexual implication of what I had done. But, I did accomplish my goal.

Janelle M. Spears, RN-C
Albany, Oregon

"Take your work seriously but yourself lightly."
~ C.W. Metcalf

Don't Bury Me In A Cheap Casket

I work in an outpatient clinic and have a close rapport with many of the patients. They often tell me their life stories and how things are going for them personally.

One patient, Cheryl, told me she was frustrated with her diet as she was not continuing to lose weight. She followed her diet precisely but just couldn't lose weight as she had been doing. I explained that she may have reached a plateau and would lose inches during that time frame before continuing to lose weight again.

The reason for her diet is the interesting part – it started as a joke between her sister and her. One day Cheryl told her sister she wanted to buried in a cheap casket. Her sister replied, "Cheryl you know we won't be able to be buried in a cheap casket." "Why?" asked Cheryl. Her sister replied, "We are both overweight. Can you see them carrying our cheap casket and it breaks apart? We have to have an expensive casket."

So I continued to encourage Cheryl – at 70 years of age – to continue on her weight loss regimen!

Janet Tally, RN
Terrell, North Carolina

"Do not take life too seriously. You will never get out of it alive."
~ Elbert Hubbard

His Pecker Got Him In Trouble

Ijumra limped into my office on Roi-Namur (one of the Marshall Islands) one day with a foot so swollen he had to slowly push his flip-flop ahead, step by step. It was obvious he would not be able to wear his steel-toes safety shoes for work today or any of the next few days.

Ijumra's foot was hot and red with a pus-filled core. Just placing a little pressure on the area drained more than ½ cup of exudates. We soaked the foot in our routine solution of betadine and water, established an intravenous line, and began our protocol-driven antibiotic treatment for this type of wound.

I called the doctor on duty 50 miles away and advised him of Ijumra's condition. Knowing the patient lived on an island without electricity or running water had me making the recommendation that Ijumra be hospitalized for enforced hygiene after debridement. The quickest route to the hospital that day was by helicopter.

While awaiting transport, I inquired, "How did this happen?" In broken English Ijumra said, "Several days ago I was eating my rice (since his home has no furniture he was sitting on the floor to eat) and this old rooster kept trying to get my food. I kept kicking him away with my foot. Pretty soon he got mad and pecked my foot."

Ijumra stayed at the hospital for over three months as they worked to save his foot from amputation. Several months later he walked into my clinic with a big broad toothless grin, and no limp!

This was truly a case where Ijumra's pecker got him in trouble!

Pamela Rodkey, RN
Medford, Oregon

The Enema Sagas

It was 1964 when I first entered nursing. Things were different then as far as on-the-job training went. I had two weeks for training and orientation. I felt better prepared than most as I brought with me the "home training" my mother gave me. I quickly learned that it is better to have "real" hospital training. When I first started giving enemas, I followed my mom's example. She would go to the bathroom, sit on the toilet, and administer her enema. Seemed simple enough. I thought this must be the right way to assist my patients in this endeavor.

So entered my first patient needing an enema. As fate would have it, he was a fireman preparing for surgery. I had not anticipated the multitude of problems that would arise from this adventure! First, I was not able to see where to place the end of the tubing – since I had told him to sit on the toilet! He had to endure the torturous "poking" before I found the right spot. I breathed a sigh of relief - which was short-lived. I learned, the hard way, that when you put the water through the tube one should raise the container slowly. Of course I put the water container sky high and tried to induce the water all at once. Water squirted all over as the tube flew out and I had to reinsert it. Cut to 20 minutes later. I finally finished the task and spent another period of time cleaning the mess in the bathroom! I told the patient that I was thankful he was a fireman for at least he was used to having water everywhere he worked! I told my supervisor about the problems I had encountered. She told me next time I was to give the enema while the patient was in bed on his left side. Imagine that! I immediately visualized the next mess that I would be getting myself into!

The next enema brought about a different type of challenge. I had a pregnant patient, who happened to be deaf, needing to be prepped for delivery. I was confident this time because I knew sign language. Unfortunately for me I would soon find that the patient understood American Sign Language. I could sign in English Sign Language. Just as unfortunate for all involved was that the patient didn't know the term "enema". I worked for about 20 minutes explaining what she was going to have done and thought she had a firm understanding. When I brought in the "bucket of water" her eyes grew big and there was a gasp of surprise. She apparently still didn't understand what in the world she had to do to get that water inside of her and why it was necessary. Ten minutes later I finally got her turned on her left side, but she didn't understand the term "hold it". Another mess was in store for me to clean.

Janella M. Spears, RN-C
Albany, Oregon

"Panic plays no part in the training of a nurse."
~ Elizabeth Kenny

Will The Real Parents Please Stand Up!!!

There must have been a full moon that night in the Emergency Department (ED). Patients were hanging from the ceiling and an intoxicated mental patient had our only doctor in a full nelson and was blubbering out her life story. I believe every ambulance in that small town was running full speed when suddenly one of the ambulance crews came bursting through the door with a young woman on a stretcher. She was moaning loudly and obviously in severe distress. A doctor's wife who happened to be visiting the ED exclaimed that someone had better hurry up and get the woman into the room because there was blood on the sheets. I ran into the room to assist the patient. In my young career, I was not prepared for what I saw next. When I pulled back the sheet there it was! A baby! Only the head was showing. The baby was blue and the umbilical cord was wrapped around its neck. I exclaimed to the mother, "You've had a baby." She immediately exclaimed, "But it's not mine. I'm not pregnant!"

Well, I was no obstetrical nurse but I had done my OB rotation and I guess instinct just kicked in. There was no time for idle chit-chat as to who was pregnant and who wasn't! I quickly removed the cord from around the baby's neck, cleared her nose and mouth with a nasal syringe, and began mouth to nose/mouth resuscitation. Between breaths I called out for help! The doctor was still in the death grip of the mental patient but after hearing the urgency in my voice, apparently freed himself. Another nurse called for an OB nurse and an isolette. Both nurse and doctor arrived quickly and took over. By that time the baby was pink and just screaming her head off. Talk about an Apgar of 10 in 0-10 seconds!

The story does not end there; however, the ED doctor went to the waiting room to congratulate the new father. In the midst of a packed waiting room, after being told about the birth of his beautiful new baby girl, the husband loudly exclaimed, "But I'm sterile!" I am told the noisy waiting room became so quiet you could hear a pin drop. The next scene I witnessed was the wife being pushed out of the ED on her stretcher with her husband walking next to her; both appearing in a state of shock. The OB nurse was walking hurriedly ahead of them pushing the new baby girl in her isolette.

Faye Miller

New York

"Humor is a spontaneous, wonderful bit of an outburst that just comes. It's unbridled, it's unplanned, it's full of surprises."
~ Erma Bombeck

Telephone Bloopers

- Working for a behavioral health managed-care company, we always answer the phone "Behavioral Health". On slow weekend shifts the staff frequently strikes up conversations between calls. In this particular business, one becomes adept at sustaining conversations with frequent interruptions. One particular day the topic of conversation between a co-worker and me happened to be religion. My co-worker was in mid-sentence when his phone rang and he promptly answered with "Muslim Behavioral Health".

- Managed care nurses who conduct business telephonically are familiar with the complexities of spelling out words and names over the phone. Upon providing referrals for participating providers to a member seeking treatment for bariatric issues, my coworker had the need to spell out a provider's name. Without forethought he came to the letter "H", which he closely followed with "as in heavy". That was followed immediately by a pause of embarrassment!

Kathy Graham, RN, MS, CARN, CMCN
Harrisburg, Pennsylvania

"Laughter is a tranquilizer with no side effects."
~ Arnold H. Glasow

The Rambling Tale
Of An Antique Nurse

- My official student nurse experience began in the summer of 1968. My years as a student nurse were the transitional years. Students were all single women. In my junior year you could get married, but banned from living in the dorms, even if the husbands had been called away to war. Why? Our best guess was they had had sex!

- The first bed bath I gave. He was a 19-year old Georgia Tech football player. His mother came in just in time to "finish the bath". Listen up wherever you are today, "You were gorgeous and could never have been more embarrassed than I was that day! Even at my current age I still regret your mother's untimely entrance!"

- My first code. "I lost my cap, where the . . . . did my cap go? And where did all these people come from?" They pushed me right out of the room. Thank God!

- My philosophy on God: I guess the most memorable fact I learned as a student nurse and continue to learn as I practice is: I do my best but am not the boss of who lives or dies. I believe there is a God since lots of my patients have survived and continue to do so....and so do I.

Elise Ledbetter, ARNP
Atlanta, Georgia

"It's easy to make a buck. It's a lot tougher to make a difference."
~ Tom Brokaw

Here Fishy Fishy

I have been a nurse for 15 years. I was working in an Emergency Room when this story took place. A female patient underwent a procedure requiring the use of Versed and was beginning to wake up. I was by her side to ensure her safety and monitor her condition. I also happened to be wearing a scrub top featuring cartoon fish. The patient stared at my shirt and while I was performing my assessment, she reached our repeatedly toward my shirt. "I almost got it", she would exclaim as she took another swipe through the air. I wasn't sure what was going on at first, but after a couple of near misses, I understood – she was fishing.

I told her to wait a minute and I got closer to her. As she grabbed, I held out my shirt and she "caught" a fish. She looked perplexed. I smiled and told her that medication was causing her to think the fish on my shirt were real. She looked at me and laughed. A few days later I received a card with a photo of a kitten dipping its paw into a fishbowl; yet never being able to reach the fish. Inside the card one word – "Thanks".

I save all the cards, notes, and letters of my patients who have been thoughtful enough over the years to send them. I take them out on rainy days whenever I feel like a cog in the medical wheel.

Patti Hoffman, RN
Anchorage, Alaska

"You grow up the day you have your first real laugh – at yourself."
~ Ethel Barrymore

At Your Service

I was coming out of the ladies room. There was an elderly woman attempting to enter the room. Her husband had pushed her – in her wheelchair – right up to the door. But the door was not automatic. She was trying to push the door open – half sitting/half standing – in her chair. That's when I pulled open the door.

I caught her by the arm and asked if she needed any help. She simply replied, "Yes." I said I would help and took her hand. I held onto her as we made our way to a stall. I took her right to the toilet. Not wanting to take any chances, I made sure she was holding onto the support bars in the stall before I stepped out to hold the door closed. I told her to call when she was ready to come out.

When she called I assisted her to the sink to wash her hands and retrieved paper towels for her. I even threw them away when she was finished as I didn't want her to have to do anymore than necessary.

On our way out of the bathroom she said, "This is such a lovely service. Do you just stand here and do this for everyone?" I said, "Yes, I do it for everyone."

Lori Wheeler, LPN
Denver, Colorado

"Comedy is simply a funny way of being serious."
~ Peter Ustinov

Is My Hair Purple?

As a school nurse, I had the opportunity to accompany an 8th grade class to a local museum. After boarding the bus and beginning the journey, I noted a small gaggle of girls who kept turning around and looking at me as if my hair was purple or my blouse was undone. They were giggling and I could tell there was something of major interest on their minds that involved me. Since my hair was (and still is) brown and my blouse was securely buttoned, I asked them if they needed something. At this question, they giggled louder and acted as if I were speaking Japanese. Now I identified the problem: one of them had a burning questing about sex.

The week prior to this trip, I had finished an education unit on sex with the 8th grade. The topic was sexually transmitted diseases. For those of you unfamiliar with this type of teaching, the class can never be long enough to cover the topic and the long question and answer sessions that invariably follow. I find that everyone even adults, are generally curious about the topic of sex. I feel it is normal human nature. Teenagers today are confused and bombarded with sexual messages, peer and cultural pressure, and misinformation. Some become extremely lost when it comes to making positive decision regarding sex.

As we progress through the tour of the museum, I noted the group of girls purposely drawing closer and closer to me. I began a casual conversation about the exhibit and they all pretended to be very interested in my words of wisdom. It was then that I asked one of the girls if they had thought of any questions from the information I gave out in class the previous week. That's when things got interesting. I received an immediate response of "Go ahead Emily; ask her." Then a second girl said "She will tell you if it is true; she knows." Now I was really curious. Finally after a bit more prodding from her friends Emily asked me: "Is it true that....you know...down below on boys....that if the sperm doesn't have a chance to come out...that you know.....their balls will turn blue and like explode?" To add to this Emily inquired "And is it really painful?"

At this point all of the girls' faces looked liked a group of deer that had been caught in the headlights. There was an awkward moment of silence as I thought of where to begin my answer. I calmly put my arm around Emily and told all the girls that testicles will not explode. I invited the girls to have lunch at my office the next day since the museum didn't seem like the best place for this conversation. I had the distinct feeling that one of the girls was getting pressure from one of the boys to do something she was neither willing nor ready to do. I followed up with them the next day and resolved their questions.

I think this is just one example of how important it is for a teenager to have someone to trust and talk to about sex. Who better than the school nurse? I love my job and feel like I really make a difference everyday. Some days are funnier than others!

Cathy Cero-Jaeger, RN, MS
Milwaukee, Wisconsin

5

Simply
Inspirational

"Rose-colored glasses are never made in bifocals.
Nobody wants to read the small print
in dreams."

~ Ann Landers

Life Lessons As Taught By Paul

I am passing along a story that I wrote and presented at one of my student's funerals during the 2006-2007 school year. Paul was an awesome little guy with severe cerebral palsy. I know we aren't supposed to have favorites as nurses (or parents for that matter), but Paul was in fact my favorite student. He was wheelchair bound and fed by a G-button. He died unexpectedly during the night after attending school the previous day. My reason for writing *Life Lessons as Taught by Paul* was to make sure his parents and family understood how important he was to those who knew him at school. They needed to know that we were grieving and it was not business as usual. I also wanted them to know Paul inspired us to be better people. He did all of this without ever saying a word; but just by being. I don't know many walking, talking, fully functional people who could ever inspire me the way this one "handicapped" child did. Makes me wonder who is really handicapped.

FUNERAL SPEECH: I had been married for a number of years prior to my arrival at Washington Elementary. Upon my arrival I fell deeply in love. Usually I go for the cerebral types, but this time I found me a charmer. Paul was his name and although he was too young for me I pursued his affections daily. Like anyone in a serious pursuit, I found out what Paul liked. His interests were varied; which only added to his renowned charm. He preferred Cool Whip to regular frosting and was partial to salad bar pudding. Shania Twain was his favor singer and had she ever recorded "The Wheels on The Bus" or "When You're Happy and You Know it" Paul would have been shocked if they hadn't gone straight to number one on the charts. Now who couldn't love a little man with taste like that?

Now I'm sure there are people who, in their narrow views, believe Paul lived a short and unfulfilling life. I would challenge that notion.

It is true that Paul's physical abilities were limited, but what kind of humanity are we if we don't believe we are more than the bodies we inhabit? I believe it is more important to focus on a person's abilities rather than disabilities. Paul's abilities were innumerable, but it is important that I point out a few of the obvious ones. He loved unconditionally and had an innate ability to appreciate life's small pleasures. A soft lap in a rocking chair with a good book was about all he needed.

Paul had the ability to make friends and keep them. A number of years ago he was in my daughter's kindergarten class. She spoke of Paul often and his was the first Valentine out of the box. Paul had legions of friend both young and old and I would like to think this is a legacy that will live forever.

Speaking of which, I read a quote recently (although I can't recall where) that read, "We all die. The goal isn't to live forever. The goal is to create something that will." Paul did this in spades just by being our Paul.

Lori Mudd, RN
Atlantic, Iowa

"The true tomb of the dead is the heart of the living."
  ~ Jean Cocteau

The Art Of Communication

I was taught in nursing school the importance of communicating with my patients; even those who are comatose or unable to understand the spoken word.

While working in an ICU, I was privileged to care for Mrs. Smith. She had the misfortune of developing a Staphylococcal infection in an open heart surgery wound. The infection was catastrophic. The patient was comatose but not on life support. Her physical care was the same every night; to include 30 minute dressing changes. During the dressing changes and throughout the night I would talk to Mrs. Smith as if she could hear me. I explained everything I did as if she were alert and could understand. If I had to move her or do something that might be painful, I explained those procedures in advance, just as, I'm sure, we were all taught to do. I told her what day it was, what time it was, if it were a holiday, and talked about how happy her family would be when she was better. Her prognosis was poor but every night I encouraged her to stay strong and that she would be alright. I did not know for certain if she would be alright, but in my heart believed she would. I prayed for her recovery. I desperately wanted her to believe in her recovery too so that she could remain strong in light of such devastating circumstances.

One night, after many, many nights of caring for Mrs. Smith in the same manner, I walked into the ICU to begin my shift and there was Mrs. Smith looking wide awake, alert, and sitting in a chair. This was a sight that I had waited a long time for. I spoke to her and she spoke back but said nothing more until I came to perform her care. I spoke to her as I had always done.

All of a sudden she looked me directly in the eyes and said, "I know you! You have been here every night. I heard every word you said. You told me to stay strong and that I would be alright. You were the voice in the darkness that made me want to continue to try to get better."

Mrs. Smith did get better and was able to go home. I believe that we must never forget to follow the basic principles and practices of nursing: even in the face of disparity. Always remember those "little things" that were taught in Nursing 101 – things that my have seemed very insignificant at the time. The human touch – the milk of human kindness – can never be replaced by a machine, a scientific study, or an antibiotic.

Alice Harris, RN

St. Louis, Missouri

"The most important thing in communication is to hear what isn't being said."

~ Peter F. Drucker

Kindness Begets Kindness

I once witnessed the most beautiful death. An 88-year old woman had no family and felt alone. She had a large Victorian home and opened it up to three female college students. They lived there for free in exchange for caring for her and her home. They became like family and when her time came, she was surrounded by the three girls – one on the right holding and stroking her arm, one on the left doing the same, and the third stroking her head and hair. All were saying how much they loved her and how much she meant to them. The woman died in the Emergency Room; both calm and peaceful, and surrounded by love.

Laura Kleeman, RN
St. Louis, Missouri

"The dead take to the grave, clutched in their hands, only what they have given away."
~ DeWitt Wallace

Fit To Knit

While working as a nurse manager on a forensic mental health unit my duties included planning, interviewing and hiring staff, and sitting on a variety of nursing committees. Although I missed direct patient nursing, I enjoyed using my experience and knowledge to further nursing and found it a challenge to solve management problems.

I continued to miss interaction with the patients and asked myself how I could change this. My schedule did not permit hours away from management duties to mingle with patients, and I set out to find a therapeutic activity I could do one or two hours a week with patients. I am a knitter, and I recalled an article from one of my magazines about the introduction of knitting in a prison. Why not the same for our forensic security unit?

I approached Jack, one of the recreational therapists, with the idea and we partnered on the venture. We discussed the pros and cons and realized our biggest obstacle was how to plan knitting for patients in a high security unit. We knew that long straight needles would not be approved so we decided upon the 16-inch circular needles. We established a protocol that each patient needed to be approved for the class by his individual therapy team, be on no restriction, and be willing to stay for the full hour each week. All needles and yarn would be counted before and at the end of the sessions. Jack and I researched men and knitting and created posters showing men from sailors to Native Americans knitting. We presented the idea at a community meeting with the patients. Five men signed up and were all approved for our first session.

Jack and I were amazed at the enthusiasm of the participants, and each had his own style. One was meticulous, with his sense of color and design immediately apparent, while another patient began a baby cap for a grandson soon to be born. Although this man had had no contact with his family for years he completed the cap and sent it. When he received a picture of his grandson in the cap he proudly showed it to everyone.

Initially, the men concentrated on learning to knit and purl. This allowed Jack and me to assess the patients for hand tremors, concentration, and the ability to follow directions. As the men gained trust and confidence, they began to talk with us and each other. Many recounted stories of grandmothers who had knitted. The flow of knitting appeared to sooth anxiety and created a relaxed environment. There was laughter about errors. Experienced knitters would share their experiences with new patients who were frustrated and ready to toss the needle and yarn.

Other staff members joined in and volunteered to hold knitting groups on the weekends. I looked forward to going to the knitting groups and hearing the enthusiasm of the patients. They loved to describe their projects and showed sincere appreciation for the staff members that held the groups on the weekends.

I left the hospital for a period of three years. When I returned I entered an elevator one day and heard a patient remark, "She taught me to knit when I was on the Frontier Unit." Talk about feeling like you have made a difference!

Carolyn Decker, MEd, RN
Corvallis, Oregon

"The most important things in life aren't things."
    ~ Quoted in bulletin of The First Christian Church of Fairfield, Illinois.

Population Explosion

What a day this has been! Twelve babies were born today in our little hospital in the middle of the ocean. To most facilities prepared for the delivery of babies, twelve may seem like a small number. But our ten bed hospital, with three nurses on duty, on a small (less than one square mile in land mass) Micronesian Atoll twelve was a great deal! This atoll, Kwajalein, 2,500 miles southwest of Honolulu and had never experienced such a population explosion.

Gratefully, one of us was an experienced labor nurse (extraordinaire); one was an experienced emergency room nurse from a rural community who had had her share of impromptu delivery experiences; and me... with critical care and postpartum experience.

One by one our local ladies quietly delivered their babies. All had experienced birth before and gratefully no two babies came at the same time. This allowed our labor nurse to work each labor and delivery individually, and then pass their care to me while the ER nurse cleaned, bathed, and examined the newborns. This rhythm of care was soon labeled the "Birthing Tango" as we became giggly with the exhaustion of our delivery marathon.

As the mothers recovered, I prepared the bassinets for occupancy. By the third baby we had run out of bassinets. With limited supplies, drawers were pulled out of desks; bath blankets tucked into them, and were readied to receive the newest member of the community.

While the moms napped and the babies suckled, we settled into documenting our day's work. Twelve babies in twelve hours and five hours of charting!

Pamela F. Rodkey, RN
Medford, Oregon

Looking Right Through

During my commutes to and from work, I constantly drive by the homeless living in our community. I see filth and trash littering our streets and public parks. I see people who seem to look right through me when they look toward me. I see children, elderly, and many who look unhealthy.

I had some spare time and decided it was time to give back to the community. I did so by joining a friend who feeds the homeless. On a beautiful sunny weekday, my husband and I drove past the homeless and past the trash littered streets to a small parcel of land. There I became part of an assembly line helping to fill Styrofoam containers with hot rice, cabbage, and pork. Then we loaded vehicles with these meals and off we went to the various homeless campsites. The homeless knew the vehicles by sight and we were soon surrounded by the old and young alike.

As we handed out hot meals, I looked into the eyes of the very people who I thought had previously looked right through me. Their eyes were alive, they smiled, they thanked us, and they blessed us. One young girl, who looked to be about 17 years old, was about six months pregnant. I couldn't help but wonder if she had even seen a doctor and if she was eating properly. How uncomfortable it must be for her to sleep on the ground. I saw a man in a wheelchair. One of the workers took his meal to him. Why was he in the chair? Any decubitis? What about infection or poor circulation in his lower limbs? One homeless lady gave one of the volunteers a hug. My initial reaction was yikes; lice, scabies, and possible infection! When did she bathe last, wash her hands in warm water, or use soap? Then the same homeless lady smiled and looked at me and said, "Thank you and bless you. It must have taken a really long time to prepare this food." To say that I was humbled and ashamed is an understatement.

Perhaps, just perhaps, it wasn't the homeless that looked at me and even through me. Perhaps it was that I just didn't really see them. Part of being a nurse is to openly and enthusiastically embrace the service role and this includes service within the very community in which we live. We have the unique opportunity to be positive role models within our own communities. Let's not just think about it, let's do it.

Penny Morrison, MS, RN

"Never look down on anybody unless you're helping him up."
~ Jesse Jackson

Where Did My Patient Go?

In 1996, while working a temporary RN job on a medical-surgical floor, I encountered what I initially believed to be a gruff old man. He was exceptionally difficult to please - or so I thought at the time.

I was taken aback by his angelic beard, peculiar smile, and his ability to know what I was thinking at times. He had several art pages in front of him, a pair of scissors, and reams of paper. He was cutting and maneuvering his papers, fumbling at times, but always focused on what I was doing in the room.

After several trips to the room, I asked him if he liked art, what his hobbies were, and such to make conversation. He briefly smiled at me, let me know that he was in a true moment of enjoyment, and when back to, "Hey, would you get me some more water? I can't take my pills without it you know." I would gladly leave the room to retrieve his water. At the end of my shift that day, I checked on him before going home. He was cozy and tucked in for the night. All was well…or so I thought.

I returned to work the next day and asked the nurse going off shift, "So how is Mr. X?" She said, "I'm not sure what you mean; there was no one here by that name." I looked at my patient list from the previous day and saw his name on it. I showed it to my colleague. Again she said, "Honey, are you sure you have the right name?" He simply wasn't there. No one knew of him. I couldn't believe it. Where did my patient go?

As I passed the front desk later in the day, the receptionist stopped me and said, "Hey Theresa, somebody left this at the desk for you." I proceeded toward her and she handed me the most intricate and finely cut three dimensional angel ornament. It was white with a string attached to hang it and on the inside had an inscription that read: "To my angel here on earth. Thank you for being my nurse."

I still have the ornament and will never know what it all meant. But I understood that day that no matter where you are or what you do as a nurse, you touch many lives. Sometimes even angels.

Teresa Renee' Betschart, RN
Longview, Washington

"I've seen and met angels wearing the disguise of ordinary people living ordinary lives."
~ Tracy Chapman

No Plain Jane

Many years ago, I was working in an open heart ICU and my patient had suffered a stroke during surgery. It happened to be a holiday and her prognosis was not good. She looked bad and had no response other than to pain. Both her family members and the doctor were depressed about the situation. As the family turned to leave, I asked a question that came out of the blue. To this day I honestly don't know why I asked it. "What was the name she was called when she was a child?" The family members looked at me dumb struck and asked, "How did you know to ask that question?" They went on to explain that she had changed her name just six months before from "Jane" to "Giselle". They then went home.

I continued with my neurological checks all night and called her name, "Jane, Jane" at every opportunity. I kept thinking of a child being called home from playing outside late in the evening. Within a few hours she began responding and soon could follow verbal commands. I called her physician at home just to say, "I thought you might want something to add to your thank you list today." There was a long pause and he said, "Estelle, when you take care of my patients they get better."

This is one of my favorite stories about trusting intuition no matter how weird it seems. I remember this story to remind myself of the amazing power of nursing.

Dr. Estelle Codier, RN, MSN, PhD
University of Hawaii, Manoa Honolulu, Hawaii

"The mark of a true professional is giving more than you get."
~ Robert Kirby

Steven

As a nurse, I have the opportunity and privilege of working with the homeless and disenfranchised. One day, as I was leaving my office, Steven arrived.

Steven had recently been diagnosed with hypertension and wanted me to take his blood pressure. When I asked what medications he was taking Steven changed. He told me he had recently been hospitalized and expressed to me that he had no desire to live any longer. He inquired, "How would you feel if you were told to get out whenever you entered a room or store? Would you want to live if you had no place to go and no one to talk with?"

Steven went on to tell me that he could not take his medications because they made him have to urinate frequently and there was no place for him to go to the bathroom. In addition, Steven was barely able to see as he was in need of cataract surgery. He was afraid of being on the streets and afraid of the police. We talked for a long time and I told Steven that I would help if possible. He told me I was the only person that had listened to him and for that he was grateful.

I related Steven's story to an associate and researched to find that that a local eye clinic donates services to low to no income people. Later that year, Steven had cataract surgery and was again able to see. The staff found living space for Steven on a nightly basis; except for the weekends. We worked with the local housing authority and Steven was interviewed. It was determined that Steven would qualify for housing. Steven was granted an apartment the following year and has been there since. Steven took the steps to become Catholic and this past Easter we all celebrated Easter mass and communion with Steven.

Steven is a changed person. He volunteers every day and no longer speaks of wanting to end his life. He is in the process of applying for Social Security Disability. I take Steven's blood pressure and keep a record for him. Because of the help he received, Steven is able to see, take his medications as ordered, and have his own apartment. This is a working example of how taking time to listen and start the process of finding resources can save one person at a time.

Sharon Christenson
Oregon

"There are many in the world who are dying for a piece of bread, but there are many more dying for a little love."
~ Mother Teresa

Grandpa

He was an old man; a body covered with some sheets and a blanket. Not a soul around to share any time that was left, a kind word to speak, or just to hold his hand. He was shoved into a corner room at the end of the hall to live out his last moments in the desolation of loneliness.

I was coming on for the 11PM – 7AM shift on the Psychiatric ward and the staff at the nurses station was reading magazines and telling jokes. They used one hallway for the patients that had mental health issues and the other hall for people who didn't fit the medical or surgical floor. The second hallway was filed with patients left to die with no families or no one to claim them.

I was doing my first rounds of the shift to make sure everyone was comfortable, asleep, or resting. When I walked into his room, I sensed his loneliness, a need for someone to be there. His breathing was slow and labored, his pulse slow and irregular, and he felt cool to the touch. He was comatose, but there was something about him that drew me close. I held his hand and felt the softness of the air as he breathed. Sensing that he just needed words of comfort and with the thought of I'm not the right one for this, I escaped. Where was his family? Why wasn't there anyone who cared about him? Why was he put here on this floor where the people were callous with no thought of kindness?

He drew me back about an hour later when I checked on him again. Sensing more urgency, I took a leap of faith. I lightly grabbed his hand and spoke softly to him, "Grandpa, Grandpa, everything has been taken care of and you can rest in peace now. All is well here and you are going to a better place. God be with you and may the angels guide you home." I stood there a little while longer and felt an overwhelming sense of peace. I had been fighting the challenge to become an RN, thinking that I wasn't cut out for the job and all the responsibilities the job would entail. I had a life and death crisis of my own at home with my son and wasn't sure which way to turn. In those moments with "Grandpa" I knew that God had my life in His hands and that the peace I was feeling would guide me through the trials I would face as I journeyed through the next years of my life.

"Grandpa" died peacefully just after I spoke with him. I did not feel or see his spirit leave but felt the sense he was at peace. Those moments with him, a stranger in a cold place, have been a source of strength for me since.

I have a passion for caring for the ill and dying but also believe in comfort for their souls. Whether they live or die my prayer will be, "May they remember a kind word, the gentle touch of a cool washcloth on a fevered brow, and the words May God Bless you".

Joyce Olson, RN
Lafayette, Colorado

"There is a time to let things happen and a time to make things happen."
~ Hugh Prather- *Notes on Love and Courage*

Rapport

I worked in an ambulatory office with parents of children with disabilities. One set of parents, with whom I had developed a long term relationship, were the parents of a 5-year old child called Ned. Ned was diagnosed with Cerebral Palsy (CP) and suffered from frequent generalized tonic-clonic seizures that his neurologist was trying to stop with aggressive multiple anti-seizure medication changes. His mother and I spoke frequently about her difficulties caring for a multisystem problematic child with so many special needs.

One Saturday afternoon I was working as a float nurse in a local hospital and saw Ned's mother. I asked her if she were here with Ned and she told me she was here with her older daughter who had just been diagnosed with leukemia. The child had had no history of any health problems. Ned's mother told me the minister of her church told her that prayer was the only treatment her daughter needed. Mom was a caring, loving, thoughtful, and wonderful person. I was surprised that she and her husband were opting against the recommended chemotherapy. I asked her a question about her church's view of treating Ned's seizure disorder with medications. She said the church understood that medication for epilepsy was necessary. I then told her a story that many of you have heard before.

There is a prayerful man stuck in a flood and he notices the water is quickly rising around his house. He goes to the second story of the house. Soon a neighbor comes by in a boat telling the man to get in and get to higher ground. The man states, "The Lord is going to save me from this flood. I do not need your help." The water rises to the rooftop and the man is clinging to the chimney when firemen come by with another boat. The man again states, "The Lord will save me." The firemen argue with the man but to no avail – they can't get him into the boat. He finally climbs up on a tree branch and is clinging to it when a helicopter comes and the pilot drops a rope for his rescue. He waives the helicopter pilot off saying, "The Lord will save me. I do not need the life line." Soon the man drowns. He gets to the pearly gates of heaven and asks, "What happened Lord? I thought you would save me." The Lord replies, "My son I sent you two boats and a helicopter; why didn't you accept my help?"

Ned's parents listened intently and realized that the help for their son included medications. Their daughter deserved medications to fight her disease as well. The doctor soon had two signatures on the consent for care form. Ten years later, Ned's sister is a beautiful young teenager who has been in remission for years from her leukemia. Nurses who develop caring mutual relationships with families will, overtime, see beneficial results.

Ruth Neal, RN
Atlanta, Georgia

"In faith there is enough light for those who want to believe and enough shadows to blind those who don't."

~ Blaise Pascal

I'm Only Human

Anyone who works in labor and delivery will testify that there can be many sad moments; as well as funny and happy ones. Luckily, the funny and happy ones are far more frequent than the sad.

It was a dark stormy night and it seemed like every pregnant woman in the city was trying to have her baby! I was working the 11-7 shift, of course, and every birthing room, high risk room, and triage room was filled to capacity. We were triaging and laboring patients in the recovery room. We were literally overflowing. I was in the recovery room when a patient came in. Barbara was only 32 weeks pregnant and in active labor. It has been prearranged that her labor would not be stopped, no matter what, because the fetus had been diagnosed with many anomalies, including Potter's Syndrome, and was not considered "compatible with life." Mom was almost 10 cm and delivery was imminent.

So we whisked her off on the cart to the last remaining birthing room (funny how God has a way of opening doors when you need it). Barbara progressed so quickly that she never made it off the cart onto the bed before she delivered. The Code Pink Team of highly qualified pediatricians was standing by and immediately intubated the baby and rushed her off to NICU. There they confirmed that indeed, the baby was not going to survive.

The pediatricians returned in what seemed like only minutes where they proceeded to extubate the baby. They handed her to Barbara so that she and her husband Tom could say hello, tell their baby how much they love her, and say goodbye. Tom sobbed so hard that not only tears, but drool was running down his face. It was at that point that I lost it. More tears than I ever thought I had came running down my face as I too, started to sob. I was so embarrassed that I called the charge nurse to the room so she could relieve me for a few moments until I could regain my composure. After all, even though nurses are generally compassionate and empathetic people, I remember being taught in nursing school that you should "remove yourself emotionally" from your patients so you don't get too involved. Boy, did I blow that one! Luckily, it seemed as though Barbara and Tom, caught up in their grief, had not even noticed me.

I went home in the morning feeling that I had failed as a nurse because I was too human. Then about a month later, I was given a copy of a letter that my unit manager had received. It was from Barbara and Tom, thanking everyone for the excellent care they received during the entire pregnancy. They thanked the doctors for helping them through the diagnosis and plans for delivery. They thanked the personnel in the Fetal Diagnostic Center and Genetics Counseling for their guidance and advice. They thanked the nurses and doctors in general who took care of them during their hospital stay.

At the end of the letter they wrote, "But most importantly, we'd like to give our special thanks to our delivery nurse, Loraine, because we know she shared our loss, and that means more to us than any words could ever say." Wow, I was floored! All that time I thought I was being a terrible nurse by not being able to retain my composure. But in the eyes and heart of my patient and her husband I was an angel!

I learned an important lesson that day. I've been a "human" nurse ever since and I buy a lot of facial tissue. To this day whenever anyone asks me what I remember most, this is the story.

Loraine Klingensmith, RNC
Ohio

Listen To Your Patient

How often are nurses reminded to listen to what the patient is telling them?

Early in my career I learned how true this pronouncement is while working the evening shift in a medical intensive care unit. The unit had eight beds and it was one of those busy nights when we were short staffed.

In mid-shift one of the patients, Mr. Goss told me he had a "stomachache". I gave scant attention to his complaint as he displayed no visible distress but he continued to mention the pain. Nearing the end of the shift, I decided I should check his dressing. Mr. Goss had undergone minor abdominal surgery and had been placed in the medical ICU due to a cardiac condition. As I removed the heavy dressing I was startled to see his bowel oozing out of an open incision on his abdomen. I quickly applied a sterile dressing and saline to the bowel and contacted the resident on call.

The resident attempted to insert the eviscerated bowel through the open incision but as he tried, Mr. Goss developed cardiac arrhythmias. It was determined the patient would have to be sent to the emergency operating room (OR). Of course at 11:30 at night it took some time to organize the OR staff. Mr. Goss was soon taken to the OR.

When I reported to work the next evening I was extremely relieved to see Mr. Goss had come through the procedure with no difficulties. But the near tragedy reinforced my resolution to always listen to what your patient tells you.

Sandra K. Sharp, MSN, ARNP
Miami Beach, Florida

Night Terror

Years ago, while still in nursing school, I worked the overnight shift at a nursing home. More often than not I was the only Certified Nursing Assistant (CNA) for the fifty residents in one wing of the facility. Some nights I was the only CNA for all 150 residents. As you can imagine, I spent the entire night going from soiled bed to soiled bed, changing sheets, and changing and re-positioning patients.

One of the women living there had night terrors. She was never able to name that which she feared, but woke every few hours screaming in panic. Her confusion and fear touched my heart as I tried to imagine experiencing her quality of life. I immediately discovered that she would calm down and return to sleep if I spent 10-15 minutes talking to her. Soon thereafter, I discovered that if I came to work 20 minutes before my shift started, held her hand, and talked with her she slept peacefully the entire night through.

Twenty minutes a day, five days a week out of the life of a student nurse was a small price to pay for her peace of mind.

JT Hayes, RN, PHN
Palm Spring, California

JT's comment: *"I believe that a large part of nursing involves giving of that of which we are made to those in need."*

"Dare to reach out your hand into the darkness, to pull another hand into the light."

~ Norman B. Rice

I Won't Give Up

Mr. Barrett was one of my home health patients. He had once been famous, traveled the world, and made a great deal of money; however, his life was much different when I first met him. He had spent his money, had very little family, and was a double below the knee amputee due to complications of diabetes. He had recently moved to town to be closer to family. He lived in a one room apartment with his dog.

I had called ahead and made an appointment to interview Mr. Barrett and get him started with his home health care. This appointment was my first clue to his personality and I wasn't wrong in my initial assessment of what I would be facing. He greeted me with a loud, "Well, come in." I found a thin man in a motorized wheelchair. The only furniture was one straight back chair and a hospital bed. He told me I couldn't sit on his bed but I could clean off the chair if I wanted to. He was also hard of hearing and yelled when he talked.

Somehow we managed to get through the interview and physical assessment. I gritted my teeth and took lots of deep breaths in order to remain calm and professional. I soon learned that tenacity would be needed to do justice to Mr. Barrett's needs. My glimmer of hope that there was more to this man than anger was the way he talked to his dog. His eyes softened and he actually talked baby talk to the little dog.

Along with weekly nursing visits, I set Mr. Barrett up for a physical therapy evaluation and contacted a prosthesis company. I finished my paperwork and felt like we were on the way to giving Mr. Barrett a better quality of life. His goal was to be able to walk again. My enthusiasm was short-lived. The first physical therapist that visited Mr. Barrett left his house in tears and refused to go back again. Luckily, Mr. Barrett's assigned nurse was tougher and he didn't scare her away!

Mr. Barrett's doctor's staff was wonderful and always went the extra mile for their patients. Of course, Mr. Barrett managed to make them all angry. There was a lot of communication with the medical clinic about Mr. Barrett's needs; his noncompliance with medications; his need for a physical therapist; and the myriad of other problems I encountered with this patient. During one of the telephone consultations with Mr. Barrett's physician, the doctor suggested that we just go ahead and discharge the patient from home health. He told me he did not see any point in continuing due to Mr. Barrett's personality; but that it was my decision. This particular doctor had worked with my office many times and had never made such a suggestion. I knew that his office staff was at the end of their rope with Mr. Barrett.

Now I had a difficult decision to make. Should I just give up on him and justify his belief that he wasn't worth being cared about? I did care for him. I still felt there was a chance to make a difference in his life. I couldn't give up on him. I decided to keep him as a patient and increased his nursing visits. We purchased a pill minder and filled it once a week. We received new prosthesis that fit him better. We even found a company that had a part needing to be replaced when his wheelchair stopped working. I begged another physical therapist to evaluate Mr. Barrett even though this wasn't her usual territory. She was tougher than Mr. Barrett and she worked with him and he started getting stronger.

I moved away, so am not sure if Mr. Barrett ever walked again. I do know that I was glad that I had not given up on him. I knew we had come a long way when on one of our last visits he asked me, "What are you doing here instead of one of my girls (his nurse and therapist)?" He told me, "I just love those girls."

Carol Skelton, RN
Pullman, Washington

"The greatest good you can do for another is not just to share your riches but to reveal to him his own."
 ~ Benjamin Disraeli

"Sometimes the best helping hand you can get is a good, firm push."
 ~ Joann Thomas

Strength Of Mind

In 2004 while working my way through nursing school I was working as a rehabilitation technician. I had a patient who had sustained a severe spinal cord injury in an automobile accident. He was completely paralyzed from the chest down, could barely raise his arms, and didn't have movement in his hands. He was unable to grip anything; making activities of daily living nearly impossible. He had no control over his bowel or bladder function. He was thirty years old with a beautiful wife and two small children.

To this gentleman, physical rehabilitation was essential in order for him to gain independence and continue to provide for his young family. With this level of injury, independence is extremely difficult to achieve. Most patients who are discharged home with this degree of injury continue to need home health assistance for hygiene and other personal assistance. As a rehabilitation technician, it was my job to teach him everything I could in order for him to achieve his goal of independence. I accepted the challenge and so began his three months of hard work.

During his stay we worked every day practicing activities of daily living; transferring in and out of bed; practicing personal hygiene, bowel and bladder care, padding, positioning, and turning in bed. He had to learn to feed himself, hold a pencil using adaptive devices, and relearn the countless tasks that most of us take for granted. There were tears some days and laughter other days! Despite his frequent frustration and fatigue, I supervised and coached him through difficult tasks instead of jumping in and doing things for him.

I see this patient today as he pulls up in the hospital parking lot in his car seat filled minivan. He comes every Wednesday for quad-rugby practice. The gymnasium where practice is held is near my office. I get to watch him speed his wheelchair up and down the court with amazing strength and energy. He is still happily married and his children are growing up. Every time I see him, I remember struggling through frustrating evenings and am so proud of him. It is so easy to give up the idea of independence with such a life changing injury. It is easy to replace determination with depression. This patient firmly took hold of the cards dealt to him and made the most of them – for himself, his family, and though he may not realize - me as well.

Jennifer Biggs, RN, BSN, CNRN
Craig Hospital
Englewood, Colorado

"Courage is being scared to death – and saddling up anyway."
~ John Wayne

Take The Time

"I'm so bored", Connie remarked as she stared at me with her jaundiced eyes and bald head. She was wide-eyed as she awaited my response. I thought about how she'd already watched nearly every movie in our DVD library and quickly offered to get her the Sunday paper from the break room. "No" she said as she lowered her head in disappointment. I was immediately aware of my lame response and annoyed with myself for missing Connie's not-so-subtle hint. In my attempt to complete my morning assessment and stay on task with my own agenda, I had missed an opportunity to respond authentically to Connie's words, which were full of anticipation. Connie had been valiantly fighting for her life and she deserved more than a newspaper.

I began to look beyond Connie's comments about boredom. Yes... she *was* bored...but that was the least of her concerns. She was not tolerating the chemotherapy well and the leukemia was persistent. This was her 108th consecutive day in the hospital for what was supposed to be a routine stay for induction chemotherapy. Instead it had cascaded into neutropenia, bacterial and fungal infections, acute delirium, ICU stays, procedures, and surgeries.

Connie was a young wife and mother of two young children. I thought back to when I first met her as she sat upright in bed with her perfect lipstick, hair coiffed, and nails painted cotton candy pink. Proudly displayed on her bedside table were framed photographs of her family. A variety of lipsticks and lotions were lined up neatly next to the picture frames along with a pretty pink address book and a vase of flowers. Although she had arrived for cancer treatment Connie made herself at home as best she could. Despite her healthy-looking appearance at the time, she had been newly diagnosed with acute myelogenous leukemia. As is common with newly diagnosed cancer patients, Connie was anxious about her treatment and prognosis. At the beginning of her hospitalization she would watch my every move and ask a multitude of questions.

As I returned from my thoughts of Connie's first days here, I sat down next to her and looked around the room. Now, months later, it was brimming with hospital paraphernalia – a bedside commode, a walker, oxygen tubing, linens, IV pumps with tubing, and multiple bags of different colored solutions. Her bedside table was no longer neatly organized with pretty lipsticks or framed photographs. It had become utilitarian; no longer useful for beautiful things or decorative knick-knacks. Today it was cluttered with an emesis basin, a water pitcher, mouth sponges, alcohol wipes, and an assortment of other necessities. As I looked up from the table I noticed the look of despair on Connie's face and began to realize that her announcement about being bored was not something I could quickly and efficiently address. It was not a simple problem or routine request that could be neatly solved in a matter of minutes. I knew this was going to take some time and was thankful that our oncology unit's nurse/patient ratio allowed for times like this.

"If you wear your mask we could take you for a walk around the hospital in your wheelchair", I offered brightly. Her face wrinkled up as she began to slowly rock back and forth, crying. "I want to go home" she sobbed. I took her hand and acknowledged her desire to go home. I asked her to tell me what she missed about home and what she would do once she got there. Always descriptive and willing to share she answered with a wet sparkle in her eyes. She described her home and family with animation and passion. I learned that Connie adored the holidays and always decorated her house from top to bottom. She was always the hostess and enjoyed making others feel comfortable in her home. These intimate details about her life were helpful in understanding her care needs, but more importantly, the talking and sharing reminded her of what she had in her family and friends.

Her posture changed from defeated to hopeful and there was a renewed calmness in her voice. At one point in the conversation she looked at me with all sincerity and asked about my home and family.

The one thing I remember most about Connie is that no matter how sick, scared, or bored she was, she always thought of others. She smiled and listened intently as I described my home and family. I noticed her body relax into the bed. Perhaps I had helped her for this short moment in her life.

During her lengthy hospital stay Connie remained hopeful about her prognosis and her potential for returning home. Hope, with its infinite possibilities, sustained her desire to be reunited with the life and home she so dearly treasured. She finally made it home for a brief period of time but was readmitted to the hospital with complications of her illness. Although she died in the hospital, we all breathed a sigh of relief that she was able to get home, even for a brief period of time, before her passing. I have been blessed by my interactions with Connie. When I think of her today I am reminded of what it means to live with compassion and to have the faith and courage to press on day after day.

Heidi Rolfs, RN, BA, OCN
Portland, Oregon

"Nurses don't wait until October to celebrate Make a Difference Day - they make a difference every day!"
~ Author Unknown

Lessons From A Mermaid

It was an unusual day in the NICU. We had several new admissions, but not the typical premature baby or meconium-stained full-term infant. This day brought new challenges.

First came Sarah, a full-term baby with growths that affected her neck, mouth, and chest. Sarah was transferred from a small hospital to our unit. During her mother's pregnancy, the doctors had noticed something was not quite right. The ultrasound revealed disturbing shadows indicating large tumor-like growths.

Sarah was a first baby and her parents were anxious for her arrival despite the warnings given by the obstetrician. So, on this day, Sarah was born by cesarean section with her father present at delivery. He watched as his daughter's grotesque features emerged from the incision. A huge growth pushed her little tongue out of her mouth, making it look like a giant blue blob protruding from her lips. Her cheeks and neck seemed to be a continuum. Huge growths misshaped her face, yet her eyes sparkled beautifully. Delicate blue eyes peering out of the fleshy mass immediately connected with her father's eyes and love was born.

Sarah's dad followed the ambulance to our hospital where the NICU staff would do what we could for Sarah. Her appearance caused some to turn away, but her eyes captured the hearts of many. We knew the growths would be an obstacle for Sarah, impeding her eating and breathing. Surgery could help, but the growths were so large they could not be removed entirely without compromising surrounding organs and tissue. Removal was going to be difficult and would not guarantee they would not grow back.

Being prepared for Sarah's appearance helped her parents and the staff bond with her and grow to love her. Her parents said, "Life gives us many gifts and they come in many different packages." Sarah was imperfect, yet a great gift.

That same day another baby was born in a small town north of the city. A frantic call came into our NICU from the staff at the small hospital. "You must come get this baby immediately! It's terrible! This baby is badly deformed."

I was the transport nurse that day, so I grabbed the tackle box filled with medical supplies--laryngoscopes, tubing, IV bags, needles— anything we would need to stabilize a sick or premature baby. The respiratory therapist with portable ventilator in hand arrived. The pediatric resident and I joined the respiratory therapist in the ambulance and we departed for the 40-mile trip. We arrived at the referring hospital to find a "mermaid" baby. Tiny, with delicate features and a beautiful face, the baby had been born with its legs fused. There were no genitalia present so we did not know the infant's gender. The baby had other defects that were not compatible with life.

We wanted to keep the child there at the home hospital, but the staff didn't feel they could take care of it. We knew it was only a matter of time before the baby would die and thought it would be best to keep it there with the family – but no one wanted the infant.

As usual, we stopped in the mother's room on the way out and asked the mother if she wanted to see the child before we left for the city. She quickly said, "No." Shortly after we got back to the city hospital, the "mermaid" baby's lungs failed and the child died in my arms.

I will never forget that day because of the lessons I learned. I learned that every baby can be loved and that any baby can be abandoned. Sarah, with her unspeakable defects, was taken in and loved by many because they were prepared for the worst but saw the best. The mermaid baby was rejected immediately after birth. People were unprepared and reacted in the worst possible way. The staff showed such disgust at delivery that the mother didn't even want to see her infant. She imagined the worst even though the baby looked beautiful wrapped in a blanket.

The gift of life truly does come in many different packages. The gifts are not always perfect or what we expect, but if we refuse to accept the gifts given, we miss something very special.

Susan Grady Bristol, RN, BSN
Omaha, Nebraska

"The heart is the toughest part of the body. Tenderness is in the hands."
~ Carolyn Forche – *The Country Between Us*

The Wedding Must Go On

There was recently a terrible car accident when a large truck had "T-boned" a car at an intersection. The car held a young couple and their two small boys. I was called to the Emergency Department to assess the mother who was 33 weeks pregnant with her third son and was currently too unstable to transfer to the OB Department. As soon as I placed my hand on her abdomen, I suspected an abruption. There was no obvious bleeding, her water had not broken, but her abdomen was painful. During the accident her seat belt had held but she has been pushed onto the center console of the car and suffered several fractures.

While assessing the patient and asking her questions, she repeatedly said that she could not stay because she was getting married the next day. I don't remember how many times she made this statement, but she continued to do so even after she was told we were moving her to the operating room. She came out of the surgery well and her third son was delivered and transferred to a tertiary center for ventilation support.

The next morning I went to check on mom and she again said this was to be her wedding day. I replied that it still could be and asked her permission to try and make arrangements. After making a few simple phone calls, a wedding was planned. Not just any wedding – a hospital wedding – complete with a wedding cake, flowers, presents, a photographer, and a minister. The entire hospital became involved in the excitement. People brought food and decorated the solarium with balloons, streamers, and fancy tablecloths. It was amazing! Family came for the wedding, as did volunteers and hospital employees from every area.

The bride, dressed in a fancy nightgown that her sister had brought in, cried. She said the wedding was better than the one she had planned. She said they had planned to go to the courthouse to be wed, but now had a real wedding!

Nancy Kuhn
Illinois

"A happy marriage is the world's best bargain."
  ~ O.A. Battista

Missionary And Visionary

I had never thought of myself as a missionary until asked to speak at the little church in Jacksonville, Maine. They had written in the weekly bulletin, *The Missionary Sharon Grant will speak of her work in Uganda.* The following was my experience as a missionary with American Hope Charities of Maine, a medical evangelical team in Kampala, Uganda in March of 2008.

The Makerere Church, where the medical team was to serve for three days, was both large and silent when we arrived. While waiting for our assignments for the day the people seeking medical assistance began arriving. The patients were quiet and sat orderly in the pews waiting for direction. Volunteers quickly ushered the waiting patients to the registration area in preparation for their clinic evaluations and exams.

I was asked to provide counseling to the women concerning healthy living practices. The women ranged from late teens to middle age and the range of educational needs was as vast as the ages of the women. Nutritional awareness, safe sexual practices, sanitation disposal, and basic education for themselves or their children were the main issues which surfaced during my counseling sessions. These identified categories only scratch the surface of the daily needs of the women I encountered.

One woman asked for advice and prayer on becoming pregnant so her husband would return and stay with her. She was HIV positive and had five children from her first husband. Her second husband wanted to have a child of his own; however, they had three spontaneous abortions and had not been able to have a child. The husband had decided to live part of the time with her and part of the time with another woman in the hopes that one of them would provide him with a child of his own. We talked of the need to have one intimate partner and use safe sexual practices. She did not appear to be concerned that her husband would become infected with HIV or pass it to other women. This woman's basic need was to have someone care for her and her children's immediate needs. Basic needs were more pressing than looking to the future, which was very bleak in her estimation. We prayed together that her husband would learn to love and respect her and would become faithful.

A young boy of five came into the clinic with his mother. He was quiet and held a cloth to his mouth. The right side of his jaw was swollen from a tooth extraction which had taken place three months prior. The swelling extended into his neck, creating a distorted shape to his face. He was provided antibiotic treatment that had been unavailable to him previously due to the cost of treatment.

A four-month-old baby was treated for breathing problems. Her mother stated that she had congestion most of the time. The child had been to the hospital three times and the family was told to bring her back for a heart scan when they had the money to pay. The baby likely had a heart defect, but without the scan the doctors in Kampala could not treat the problem. Without the money to pay for the scan the child was sent home. The mother had hoped there would be the possibility of a scan being provided at the clinic. The tiny baby was given medicine to help ease her breathing and later the funds were obtained for the scan.

A young woman with typhoid cried with me for thirty minutes. The pharmacy had no medication to treat her. One of the local doctors had asked her to come back the next day and he would provide the medication from his own practice. She did not understand how to take preventative actions for healthy living. Boiling the water she would use and sanitation needs were discussed. She was counseled on abstinence, safe sexual practices, and tested HIV negative.

These are only a sample of the dozens of people we counseled those three days at the free clinic. The people I met were friendly, eager to please, and willing to listen to the advice provided them. They needed basic hygiene education to understand the spread of disease and preventative actions. Nutrition education was an area lacking for most of those arriving at the clinic.

My experience in the free clinic at the Makerere Church in Kampala, Uganda was exciting, frustrating, emotional, and very satisfying. My part in assisting with the treatment of a young HIV positive mother and her month old baby created a desire in me to continue helping the poor and uneducated of Uganda. Taking part in the mission trip did not make me feel important or superior to the people we were treating. The experience was humbling.

Sharon Grant
Calais, Maine

For Information on how you can assist with similar mission trips, you may contact American Hope Charities Corporation directly. They are a faith-based and medical evidence-based non-profit organization driven and committed to bringing hope and saving lives one person at a time. The purpose of the medical mission is to provide access to general medical and dental health care to the poor and the needy living in the slums and rural areas of Nairobi and Kampala. The beneficiaries of their missions are orphans and vulnerable children, young people (14-23), and adults.

If you are interested in receiving more information please contact: Sharon Stevens-Grant, 21 School Street, Calais, Maine 04619 at s.grant@americanhopecharities.org

Story Of Timing And The Watch

I was 50, tired of working outside, and needing a change in occupation. While taking a math course at the university, I was told about the Department of Vocational Rehabilitation Program. With bad shoulders from being a lifelong carpenter, I qualified for the program. "What do you want to do?" "I want to be a nurse", I replied. To make a long story short, I was accepted to the BSN program at the University of Alaska.

Four years later I finished, passed the NCLEX, and was an RN. Faced with a great deal of debt, having four children to support, and being 54 years old, I wondered if I had made the right choice. My wife and I calculated we would be debt free when I was 75 years old.

A week later my wife and I decided to go to the mall to walk around. We didn't have any money so were not concerned about overspending! As we walked through Nordstrom, my wife was sidelined by a beautiful watch. She looked at it for a long time and just loved it. She then saw the price, which was $3,000, and I saw the disappointment in her face. I felt bad, feeling that she deserved the watch for putting me through the last two years of nursing school.

The next day she told me how she had prayed that the desire for the watch would leave her and her prayer had been answered. A few days later, the doorbell rang and it was the postman with a registered letter. I thought, "Oh no, we are being sued." I opened the letter, which was addressed to my wife. She looked at the letter from the Reader's Digest. The opening of the letter read, "Congratulations. You have just won the Sweepstakes worth $250,000." She got the watch.

Walter J. Liedke, RN
Anchorage, Alaska

Nursing Is Love

The Coronary Care Unit (CCU) doorbell rang near the end of my shift on an early summer evening. I checked the bright green lines that blipped across the cardiac monitor screens before I left the nursing station to answer. When I pulled open the heavy door, in the glare of the hospital corridor, stood a woman. She was trim, about 45 years old and dressed in a wrinkled dress with a light sweater tied over her shoulders. She pushed her dark hair back from her face as she shifted her small suitcase from one hand to the other. "Hi, I'm James' mom. I got here as soon as I could. How is he? May I see him?" Her voice trembled and she wore a mask of worry and fatigue on her face. I held out my hand, drew her into the dim CCU and guided her to her son's bedside. His long, narrow form was stilled by light sedation and he lay covered by a white sheet.

"James, I'm here. Mom's here now James," she said in a soft, soothing voice as she stroked his arm and squeezed his hand. His eyelids fluttered and he sighed deeply, as if relieved of all worry and tension. That was the beginning of an unforgettable three month odyssey for me as a new nurse.

It was 1969, and James, with his shoulder length dark hair and full beard, was in his early twenties. After graduating from college, he had moved from out of state to a small farm near the hospital to "live off the land" with a group of like-minded young people. He had only been there for a few months when he became ill with flu-like symptoms that worsened within hours. His friends brought him to the emergency room and notified his parents when he was admitted to the CCU. His diagnosis was endocarditis.

His condition was a challenge from the beginning. It was the proverbial one step forward two steps back. Our hopes would be raised one day and then dashed the next as James suffered through several courses of high powered antibiotics, two open heart surgeries, and weeks on a ventilator. Nothing really worked. The relentless infection and complications took him away inch by inch. We tried everything possible to save him, but as we watched helplessly, his taut muscular body wasted away, his spirit faded, the light in his eyes went dim, and he retreated into the shadowy world of the gravely ill.

Through the shiny days and light evenings of that long summer, his mother never left. She went back to her hotel to sleep, but every day and every evening she was at James' bedside, coaxing him to eat "just a bite or two"; reading to him from the books he loved; conveying the best wishes and latest news from family and friends; and reminiscing about happy family times. She was an integral part of James' care. His father flew in often to be with his beloved and only son and to support James' mother through their surreal nightmare.

When James died, his mother was holding his hand, while nurses and doctors, who had come to love James, stood silently around his bed. We had failed to save James' life, but we had done the very best we could for him. He had done so much more for us. It has been 39 years since James died and I have been retired from nursing for several years. Yet I have never forgotten James or his mother and the valuable lessons they taught me. I learned that modern medicine will never have all the answers; that the emotional and spiritual aspects of care giving are every bit as important as tasks and techniques; and most importantly that nursing is love.

Joy Dobson Way, RN, MS
Ashland, Oregon

"Nobody has ever measured, even the poets, how much a heart can hold."
~ Zelda Fitzgerald

Victoria

I just returned to my desk after attending a memorial service for one of "my" Cacoon kids. Oddly enough, it is the second service in a two-week period of time. My mind and emotions are very weary. I feel somewhat fragile but at the same time feel gratitude that I could be involved in the lives of these children and their families. It was a privilege to have a role in their lives and affirming to play a part in their end-of-life processes.

Little Victoria was only eight months old when she passed away. She taught me a valuable life lesson. She survived far beyond what was expected of her. She was born with multiple congenital anomalies; including major heart defects. Despite the poor prognosis, she went home and continued to survive through many illnesses and operations.

Her mother devoted herself to this little angel. Mom provided attentive and admirable care. She awed me with her precise knowledge of Victoria's numerous medications. She devoted herself to giving the best care that Victoria could have received. She did all this with no grasp of the English language and in a new country where she had no immediate family.

I am so grateful that with this family in particular, I had the participation of my Cacoon promotora. A promotora is an outreach worker in a Hispanic community. Gabriella supported this family in so many ways, the least of which was interpretation. She provided ongoing support from the time of initial discharge right up until the end. In fact, when Victoria passed away, it was Gabriella whom mom contacted first. She needed help simply figuring out how to claim Victoria's body. So, we embarked on an exploration of choices available to the family, including whether to seek cremation or burial in the state or transport the body back to Mexico.

I believe that my promotora helped this family ease through what had to have been the most difficult decision of their lives. She offered hugs, information, culturally sensitive empathy, and interpretation in an extreme situation.

Yes…it was difficult seeing the broken heart of this mother; however, all of the efforts felt worthwhile. I guess as professionals we never quite know what we may encounter. But I believe that we, as nurses, are uniquely gifted with a grace to help. To help with the process of living, but also with the process of helping families let go. It is so important to provide information, support, and dignity.

Laura Scheer, RN, BSN, PHN
Hood River, Oregon

"The fragrance always stays in the hand the gives the rose."
~ Hada Bejar

Never Miss A Teaching Opportunity

I was working in home health and caring for a mother of 5 children. She was in her early thirties and slowly dying of cancer. We had nurses in her home around the clock to monitor her IVs, CAD pump, and pain medications. She had a 12-year old son who had an especially close bond with his mother. With all that was going on in her life he was getting lost in the shuffle. We were asked to find opportunities where he could spend more quality time with his mother.

Like most children his age, he was into the hi-tech stuff. As I was operating the pump one day and regulating his mom's IVs I thought of him. I checked with his mother and my supervisor and they agreed that it would be okay for him to learn how to work with his mom's IV.

I took some of the tubing and an IV bag and her son and I went to the bathroom to practice getting the air out of the tubing. He did great! Next, he watched me intently as I reached down into his mother's gown and gently pulled out the end of the Hickman catheter. I then cleaned it with alcohol, closed the clamp, disconnected the old tubing, connected the new tubing, secured it with tape, opened the clamp, and set the pump again. He watched me go through the process a few times.

Then it was his turn to give it a try. As I watched over his shoulder, he did everything exactly as I had done. He was so intent and focused on the task at hand he didn't give a second thought to reaching into his mother's gown for the end of the Hickman catheter. She lightened things up by jokingly exclaiming, "Hey! Watch it Bud!"

In time, he had the technique down perfectly. This young man's dedication to his mother enabled us to eventually pull the night nurse out of the home and give some private time back to the family.

Sherrill Hawley, RN
Salem, Oregon

"Success is how high you bounce when you hit bottom."
~ General George S. Patton

My Most Memorable Case

Having worked in pediatric oncology for over 30 years I can think of dozens of patients and their families that have touched my heart and have helped me to grow professionally and personally. It is difficult to determine which one is most unforgettable to me; so in this *My Most Memorable Case,* instead of sharing one "case" I would like to take the opportunity to highlight several of the interactions and experiences that have left a profound and lasting impression on me.

Susie was an incredible 10-year-old with refractory AML whom I cared for in the early 1980's. She was assertive and often demanding and did not hesitate to tell you what she thought and made no qualms telling a nurse or resident whether or not she would permit them to try to start an IV on her or do an LP. She frequently would say, "I have to be stuck all the time, so I allow only the best to do it." At the time of what would be her last relapse, her hair had grown back and she had this terrific short mop of curls which was her pride and joy. When we discussed potential treatment options and choices with Susie and her mom, her only question was, "Will this chemotherapy cause me to go bald?" When told yes, she immediately said, "I don't want any more chemotherapy because I know that no matter what you do I will still die and I don't want to die bald." Her mother respected Susie's choice and over the next two months until her death she lived life to the fullest and the picture of this joyful vibrant girl with curly hair remains in my heart.

George was 15 at the time of his brain tumor diagnosis and he experienced every complication that you can imagine including mutisim and hyperirritability associated with severe posterior fossa syndrome. He also developed vocal cord paralysis resulting in the need to receive a tracheotomy and gastrostomy-tube as he was unable to swallow. George remained hospitalized, often in the PICU, for six months before he was well enough to be transferred to a rehabilitation unit. Over the course of the next year he was in the hospital more than out to receive chemotherapy or for episodes of fever and neutropenia. Towards the completion of therapy, George still had numerous neurologic deficits that left him dependent on his tracheotomy and being wheel chair bound, but he had recovered his enthusiasm for life and was an inspiration for other patients as well as staff. To celebrate the completion of his treatment, George asked me if I would help him plan and carry-out a surprise party for his Mom that he wanted to hold in the family room on our inpatient unit. When I asked him what was the occasion, his response was, "I've been saving my money so I can throw my Mom a party to thank her for everything she has done for me and invite all of the nurses, doctors and other hospital staff to come so they can see how much I love and appreciate her." I'm happy to say that with the help of various other team members and a donation from a parent support group (so George didn't need to use his savings) the party was a huge success and a complete surprise to his mom. More than 50 people attended including most of his nurses, doctors, and ancillary staff, as well as his step-father and siblings. George had achieved his goal of publicly demonstrating his love for his Mom.

The last person I would like to highlight is actually a sibling. Maria was 8-years-old when her 4-year-old sister Ruth was diagnosed with a brain tumor. Ruth's disease course was rapid and difficult; due to spinal cord metastases, she became paraplegic within days of her diagnosis and the family's life changed not just because Ruth had a life-threatening cancer, but because she also required complete physical care including urinary catherization multiple times a day. During Ruth's prolonged hospitalization Maria came to visit on a regular basis. Often times, when Maria was there, Ruth would be at therapy or asleep and it soon became a standing practice that when Ruth was otherwise occupied,

Maria and I would go sit out on the hospital patio to have something to drink and talk. This young girl, with the infinite wisdom of a child taught me a great deal. On the day of Ruth's death, she informed me that Ruth's death was harder for her than it was for her parents. When I asked why, her response was, "My mom and dad still have a daughter but I no longer have a sister." Another life lesson from a child; demonstrating the different types of loss that families go through.

These three examples are just a few of many memories. I'm sure that any nurse who has worked with children has similar experiences and reminiscences. Whenever I hear people say, "How do you work in such a depressing field?" I just remember the children and families who have touched my life and think of the joy and reward that being a pediatric oncology nurse has brought me.

Karla Wilson RN MSN FNP-C CPON
Duarte, California

Previously published in *APHON Counts*, Volume 2, Number 2, Summer 2008; published by the Association of Pediatric Hematology/Oncology Nurses.

"More important than a work of art itself is what it will sow. Art can die, a painting can disappear. What counts is the seed."
~ Jan Miro

Time To Fish

One of my favorite patients was completing chemotherapy for the day. Notably, he was near the end of his treatment regimen for carcinoma of the lung. He knew his situation and prognosis were not optimal. On the one hand he was very robust and liked to do everything for himself. On the other hand, he knew he had the unthinkable…he had lung cancer.

On his chemotherapy days, he related many personal stories of his life's journey. He also shared what he truly enjoyed doing in his spare time. He enjoyed spending time with his family of course but his love was fishing. He longed for the fishing days to arrive – quickly. He told me about rituals, boating processes, and bait secrets. I think a lot of the stories were told to keep me in the room during his treatments. You know, you can sense fear without hearing the words – and that's exactly what I sensed as I listened to his stories. I learned a great deal from this gentle, kind man.

This pattern continued throughout his treatments. Then the day came. He was completing treatment for the day and I was explaining the customary home care as well as reminding him of his next appointment. That's when things got serious. He looked at me and asked me in a hushed tone, "Am I going to make it until tomorrow?" I knew that despite seemingly breezing through his treatments, he remained extremely frightened. So in a serious tone I said, "I cannot be certain that any of us will make it until tomorrow. Life can be uncertain, and changes at every corner, and at this corner you were given this diagnosis. But, I am here to do the very best for you." He grinned, breathed a small sigh of relief. I continued by saying, "I *can* tell you that it appears you are breathing just fine, you are speaking just fine, you are walking just fine, etc." I asked him if he would like for me to arrange a home health nurse to assess his home. He declined. I also reminded him of accessing emergency services should he need that and that our office is only a call away. Then, he breathed a long sigh of relief.

As I write this today, this dear man is doing well. He has been off treatments for over a year and a half. He continues to fish!

Barb B. Carpenter, MSN, ARNP, FNP, CPON, AOCNP
Louisville, Kentucky

"If people consentrated on the really important things in life, there'd be a shortage of fishing poles."
~ Doug Larson

Connecting

I am a new nurse and love my work in the postpartum unit. The best part is making a difference in the lives of new parents and connecting with them in special ways. Being a mother myself, I often find common threads with my patients.

One night I was working with a family and, in particular, a mom that I felt a special connection with. This mom was having a rough emotional time. Her newborn daughter was having breastfeeding problems and both mom and baby were awake most of the night. Early in the morning mom received a call from her husband that her other child was ill. The older sibling was vomiting and upset and the dad was unsure of what to do. His fatigue added to the mom's emotional distress. I had a similar situation occur when I was in the hospital with my newborn. I knew how hard it was being in the hospital, caring for a newborn, and knowing that a child was at home is ill, sad, and both missing and needing Mommy. Mom and I cried together.

I can't describe how good it felt to connect so closely with my patient. We have physical assessments to do and medication to administer, but we must never forget our other roles are just as important! Giving a new mom the time to express her emotions, reassurance that she is doing everything right, and a hug at 3AM are just a few ways to share the important time in her life.

Christina Robledo, RN
Clackamas, Oregon

"You may give gifts without caring – but you can't care without giving."
~ Frank A. Clark

Advocate

I am the district nurse for approximately 10,000 students in the South San Francisco area. In August 2007, the state superintendent handed down an advisory to all schools in California, stating that anyone working for a school district could volunteer to administer insulin to a diabetic student. This advisory was contrary to California State Law and the California Business and Professions Codes which governs my licensure as an RN.

At about the same time, a kindergarten student was enrolled in my school who needed complete assistance in her diabetic care. In the past, either parents came to administer the insulin to their children, or the child was independent enough to administer medication to him or herself. I hoped my district would consider hiring a private agency nurse to care for this student, but it was cost prohibitive. I let the district superintendent, as well as the other administrator at our district office, know where I stood on training unlicensed personnel to administer a highly dangerous drug. I put them in the position of making an informed decision regarding the care of this little girl and students like her.

Our heath technician took time out of his daily schedule to be at this particular school each day to check the little girl's blood sugar at snack time. I completed the lunch routine of checking blood sugars and administering insulin.

The school district supported me and provided the impetus to correctly care for this little girl. Many schools in our district made adjustments to assist me to ensure I had the time to perform this duty. I feel honored they trusted my judgment enough to allow me not to follow through on the advisory and kept our students safe! It is a true example of teamwork!

It should be noted that, on October 5th 2007, the American Association of Nurses and the American Nurses of California filed a civil suit in Superior Court in Sacramento against the State Superintendent for this advisory.

Bonnie White, RN
San Francisco, California

"We ourselves feel that what we are doing is just a drop in the ocean. But the ocean would be less because of that missing drop."
~ Mother Teresa

Against The Odds

I graduated nursing school in 1981. I spent the first eleven years of my career as a nursery/NICU nurse and loved every minute of it. It was also during this time that I was fortunate enough to marry my high school sweetheart and give birth to my three daughters. I then became very ill and required a heart transplant. My brother had received a heart transplant 18 months earlier. We are the first recorded sibling heart transplants at Emory University in Atlanta.

After a two year recuperation period I started a nursing program in our local school system and implemented a program to pay for the nursing staff. My program was duplicated all over the state. I spoke at the National Superintendents' Convention and have been a part of the Georgia Association of School Nurses since its early stages. I served as a committee chair, Vice-President, and finally President of the organization. I was chosen as School Nurse of the Year in 1999. Our nursing program in Thomasville is exceptional and we pride ourselves as having a nurse in every school. Most are Registered Nurses, but we have some fantastic Licensed Practical Nurses as well.

My daughters are all in their early twenties. Each one is a well adjusted, educated, strong, and independent young woman. Our youngest just graduated from a RN/BSN program with the highest grade point average in her class. I hope they learned something from their mom who overcame the struggles of enduring a heart transplant and a career while they were growing up.

Terri Matthews, RN
Thomasville, Georgia

What Terri said that inspired me, *"Thanks for including my short story. It is amazing how so many emotions, hurt, pain, and suffering happen in life but it can be put into words in only a few short paragraphs. My brother has since died. He live for 11 years post- transplant, I have survived over 17 years now. Quite amazing!"*

122

Diligence

I am 54-years old and think back to struggling as a young mother at age 16. I quit school in December of my sophomore year (to avoid dissecting a frog), turned 16 in April of the following year, and had my daughter in July. My mother-in-law got me a job making beds at a health care facility in September. My son was born the following July. I spent a total of 6 years of my career working as a nursing aid. I grew up and my now ex-husband delayed doing so for many years. At 21-years old I was divorced and the single mother of 2 small children.

I began working at a local mill to make more money. I stayed a year before moving out of state and beginning GED classes. I was later blessed to receive grants and a loan to continue my education through a Nursing Associate Degree Program.

Being a single mom and having quit high school way too early, I had a difficult time with Chemistry. I held two jobs, one of which I got home from at 3AM, and had Chemistry class at 7AM. I ended up dropping out and figured I would never achieve my dream of becoming a nurse. Being diligent I tried again two years later. I got an A- in Chemistry and decided there was hope! I finished my nursing program with a C+ average, as I continued to work two jobs through school to make ends meet. I had no financial support from my ex-husband and my children had little emotional touch with him. Not only did I have school and finances to contend with, but my son's behavior became a constant challenge. I finished my nursing program and became an RN the summer that coincided with what would have been my 10th year high school class reunion.

I have been in health care since 1970 and an RN since 1982. I have worked surgical units, mental health, medical-surgical floors, utilization review, case management, discharge planning, infection control, and employee health. It was not easy – and I thought the two years of nursing school would never end – but looking back it went quite fast – as have the past 25 years.

I share my knowledge daily about disease prevention with the public with the hope that people will continue to take ownership for their personal health and practice prevention. This is an incredibly rewarding feeling.

So, as I always tell others, "If I can do it, YOU can do it!" Never give up and always stay focused on the light at the end of the tunnel. The long hours of study, completing loan and grant applications, and all the other trials and tribulations you experience along the way are indeed worth it! I can't imagine having done anything else.

Mary Ann Bernard, RN
Burns, Oregon

"An education is like a crumbling building that needs constant upkeep with repairs and additions."
~ Louis Dudek

Giving Back

I am an occupational health nurse. One of my duties is training first responders. These volunteers are trained in first aid and CPR in order to provide immediate emergency medical care to ill or injured employees until medically trained staff arrives. Since I live in a small farming community, I extended the first aid and CPR training to the local police and fire departments for free.

One day, one of the first responders I had trained was first on the scene of an extremely bad automobile accident. A Volkswagen had crossed the median and become lodged under the front of a semi-truck. The driver of the Volkswagen was my husband and he had died immediately upon impact. It will always comfort me to know that he was at least granted the opportunity of immediate response. It also makes me acutely aware of how much we can do for our communities if we are willing to go the extra mile and find avenues to provide our expertise.

I offer education programs on prevention and wellness for employees at my jobsite. I have been told by more than one employee of the lives changed and saved as a result of the knowledge and education I provide. As nurses we can do so much for so many! God has blessed us for choosing this profession and has given us the secret of full and happy lives.....GIVING TO OTHERS!

Sandi Thompson, RN, COHN-S, LHRM
Largo, Florida

What Sandi said that inspired me, *"I still feel we can provide our communities, friends, family, work sites, and God so much because we are nurses."*

How Do You Feel?

I was a perky new graduate and my first patient was a man with throat cancer who had neither been out of bed nor talked for more than 10 years. Being young and eager I would start every day with, "How are you feeling Mr. Smith?" There was just silence since he didn't speak.

I went about the morning bathing him and doing all the "nurse duties" and talking all the time about the weather or the day. This was the nervous chatter of a young person who doesn't know what to do when there is no response.

After two weeks of providing Mr. Smith's care I was reassigned. I walked into his room and with the same chipper enthusiastic voice of youth said, "Good morning Mr. Smith. This will be the last day I care for you since I am being sent to another floor. I am very sad and will miss you. Oh I almost forgot, Mr. Smith – how do you feel today?" Ever so slowly he started to raise his right hand. I was in shock – as he had not moved an inch in the two weeks I had cared for him.

I watched with eagerness to where the hand was going. With much effort and what seemed like an hour of time this hand was finally directly in front of my face. Then ever so slowly, he rubbed his index finger and thumb together. I laughed. I got his joke – he felt with his fingers. I swear I saw a twinkle in his eyes and almost a smile when I reacted with such glee to his answer to my question!

Carla Nierengarten, RN, BSN, NCSN
Milwaukee, Wisconsin

"There are times when silence has the loudest voice."
~ Leroy Brownlow - *Today is Mine*

Memoir Of A Teen Pregnancy

At age 17, having just started my senior year of high school, I realized I was six days late for my period. I didn't think I was pregnant. I didn't have morning sickness, an increased urgency to urinate, or food cravings. At one point, my boyfriend Lucas put his hand on my stomach which made my stomach upset. I asked him to move his hand and he jokingly asked, "What do you have an alien in your stomach?"

I remember taking a store bought pregnancy test like it was no big deal. I wasn't even nervous because I truly felt it would be negative, as I sure wasn't one of those teenagers trying to become pregnant. When the two pink lines appeared, I only remember dropping to the ground and crying. I was not crying because I was pregnant, but because of whom the father was. I kept thinking, "Why him?"

I had to tell Lucas, although I was sure he would leave me in the dust. Actually, prior to the big news, I had actually planned on breaking up with him. He was pushy, verbally abusive, and didn't have much going for him. He was 23 years old and still living with his mom. I hadn't been with him for very long. When I first met him, I just wanted to hang out. I never intended on it going this far. I told him repeatedly that I didn't want to have sex. I had been going to church and doing really well. I didn't want to do anything with him, but I felt uncomfortable saying "no" to him over and over. We didn't use a condom and I wasn't on birth control. Letting him use a condom would have meant that I was okay with it. I know now that I should have stuck up for myself and should not have been with someone like that. I later found out that he had one kid that was adopted out and another girl pregnant at the same time that I was. I also found out that he had several psychosocial diagnoses that prevented him from working. Apparently, I had picked a real winner.

I told my mom Sunday. I thought she would take it the hardest, but it was actually my stepdad that took it the worst. He has always treated me like his own daughter and was disappointed in me. They were both upset when they found out Lucas' age and to this day regret not pressing charges against him. My parents were very concerned about me graduating school. I have always liked school and I never worried that anything, including this situation, would prevent me from graduating.

Going to school pregnant was not a problem for the other kids. I was friends with just about everyone so I was never teased for being pregnant. The worst thing I remember was people staring at my belly while I carried my lunch tray. It was also difficult finding a prom dress that would fit me because I was 9 months pregnant. I gave birth to a beautiful healthy little girl named Jill in May 2001. I graduated in June with the rest of my class with my baby in the audience. I will never forget the extra loud cheer I had received from my classmates when my name was called. I was told later they were very proud of everything I had accomplished.

Statistics show that teen moms have high risk factors for having low birth weight babies and high incidents of getting into drugs and abusive relationships. I have witnessed teen moms that have had their children taken away. Luckily, I never got into drugs, had a healthy baby, and did not have Jill taken away. However, I felt stuck in a verbally abusive relationship. Her father took the news of my pregnancy surprisingly well. I had expected him to leave me, but he didn't. He did help take care of the baby by changing her diapers and bringing her to my workplace so I could feed her. As far as finances were concerned, he would constantly lose jobs and I was forced to pay for everything. When he did have money, he would spend it on his car. He cheated on me several times and was verbally abusive by calling me names and yelling bad words.

Although I felt stuck I wanted things to work out for my daughter's sake. I wanted us to be a happy little family with our own house. I wanted to go back to school and have a successful career. I thought it was never going to happen. One day, I got the best news. It was my escape. My low income housing unit, which I had applied for two years earlier, has come through and would be available in a few months. I decided not to tell Lucas.

He only got physical once; which was the night I finally left him. I called my friend at 2AM, told her what had happened, and that I was coming over. She said she had been waiting for this phone call for two years.

Living in low income housing was hard, but I was able to go back to school. I chose nursing. I saw nursing as a career where I would feel good about what I did and still be able to take care of my daughter. When I was pregnant in high school, one of the last semester classes I had taken was in the nurse's office. It was supposed to be a chance for me to rest and do homework. I realize now that the nurse was also there to monitor and educate me. I was also fortunate to have a visiting nurse for teen moms. A nurse would come once a month to weigh Jill and answer any questions. I looked forward to our visits. I got close with both nurses. We have nurses in our family and I believe that a combination of these factors motivated me to become a nurse.

Today, Jill and I are doing wonderfully. I am working as an RN and going to school earning my BSN. We just bought our first house two weeks ago. Jill has been so patient while I have been in school. I feel she has finally received what she deserved and what I had promised – a house of our own. Our neighborhood is wonderful with lots of kids for her to play with. I am with a wonderful man who treats me with respect and has similar goals to mine. As far as Jill's father is concerned, he has short supervised visits with Jill three times a year. I feel bad that she doesn't have a better relationship with him but know it is safer for her this way. She has a very strong relationship with his family. Lucas has four or five children now; all from different mothers. Jill and I have a relationship with one of the children. This child is Lucas' son and his mother is the other girl that was pregnant with Lucas' child at the same time I was. Jill has a brother and his family. As for me…I have my happiness.

Why am I telling you all this? Get to know that special someone well before making "that" commitment. Don't take the long hard road that I took. Parents, listen to your children. Be supportive no matter how hard it may be. Let your children know that they can come to you with anything; without feeling judged or put down. For teens that are already mothers, I hope that my story will encourage you to leave if you feel stuck in a bad relationship. I hope too my story will encourage you to move forward with your lives.

Hope Duncan, RN
Washington, D.C.

What Hope said that inspired me, *"Go accomplish your goals! Do it as an example to your child. If I could do it, then you can do it."*

"Good thoughts bear good fruit, bad thoughts bear bad fruit – and man is his own gardener."
~ James Allen

Wind Beneath My Wings

I had just started my shift and my patient load was unusually light. I knew all but one of my assigned patients and all were stable. One of my patients was an elderly woman named Mrs. Jannies. Her death was imminent, but she had supportive family members with her around the clock. I had worked with her for a number of days and always found her cheerful and smiling. She had told me she was quite prepared to meet her maker and was simply waiting for the right moment to be called. The only patient I had not previously worked with on the floor was Mrs. Williams: a young woman in a coma. She was in her 30s and the mother of a young daughter. She had succumbed to a severe infection that required heavy antibiotic treatment. She had complications from the antibiotics resulting in complete organ shut down and her present coma state. She had been in a coma for a number of weeks, was comfort measures only, and one could assume she was just not ready to die.

I proceeded to assess my patients starting with the acute and then onto my two ladies who were comfort measures only. I entered Mrs. Jannies' room and as expected, was greeted with a smile from the patient and her two daughters. Her eyes were alive and bordering on mischievous. She pulled out a brightly wrapped gift from her bedside table and said, "This is just for you." I politely declined, explaining that I could not accept a gift. She then reached for another identically wrapped gift and said, "I know that's why I have another just for the rest of the nurses." I graciously accepted but groaned inwardly thinking - just what I needed more chocolates. After my assessments and a brief chat I dropped off the gift for my coworkers and placed my gift in my locker. I proceeded to my last patient, Mrs. Williams. The clipboard outside of her room displayed that her vitals, recently taken by my assistant, were stable and the patient had had an uneventful night.

I entered Mrs. Williams' room to find the sheets tucked neatly around her. I could tell that my assigned nursing assistant had already been in the room as she always took great pains to make sure the sheets were so neatly tucked. Mrs. Williams didn't look as if she were dying. Her cheeks had some color and her hair…. it was out of place. She had hair covering her right eye and cheek. I slowly brushed the hair away from her face and then said something that to this day I don't know why. I said, "It's going to be okay. It's okay for you to go. Don't be afraid." Then I saw it. One single teardrop fell onto her left cheek. She had heard me! Mrs. Williams died six hours after I had told her it was okay to go.

After an emotionally draining 12 hour shift, I left the hospital with my brightly wrapped chocolates and placed the package on the passenger seat and started my long drive home. My thoughts were on the day – so much had happened. Why had I said what I did to Mrs. Williams? When I had repeated this story to the nurses on the unit they reassured me that sometimes patients simply need to be told that it's okay to go. It still did not make me feel better.

I was still reflecting on my day when I stopped at a red light. I glanced over to see the brightly wrapped gift and decided a chocolate was just what I needed. I quickly unwrapped the paper only to find that it was not chocolates after all. Instead it was a hanging ornament with the words: "You are the wind beneath my wings." Tears welled up in my eyes. Perhaps….just perhaps…. I was the wind beneath Mrs. Williams' wings….perhaps she just needed to be told it was okay to go.

To this day I have not forgotten either lady. The ornament is prominently displayed in my living room and serves as a constant reminder that there are truly times nurses are the wind beneath the wings of their patients.

Penny Morrison, RN, MS

Jazzy Jeff

I work as a public health nurse specializing in tuberculosis (TB). The patients in my clinic with TB are followed daily by an assigned case manager. We do Directly Observed Therapy (DOT). A homeless patient was screened for shelter use and found to be very ill with TB. He was a self-admitted "garbage head", meaning he drank alcohol heavily and did any drug available to him. He went by the moniker of "Jazzy Jeff" and was well known on the streets.

Jeff was violent when he was under the influence. I was able to hook him up with an agency that did outpatient drug and alcohol counseling and provided housing. He practically destroyed a room and then a house he was placed in by throwing furniture and appliances around! Jeff was also often non-compliant with his TB treatment regimen. I had to track him down several times on the streets. He was a "flyer" – a person who stands at freeway off-ramps with a sign soliciting for help. All in all – a difficult challenge in a person who required nine months of TB treatment with multiple medications. Jeff completed TB treatment during which he had short periods of being clean only to relapse. After completion, he used to come by the clinic inebriated to the point of falling down and ask the staff for money.

It is now two years since Jeff completed TB treatment. I saw him on the street recently. He's been clean and sober for over a year, has stable housing, and a real job. He looked healthy and thanked me for being one of the catalysts in his recovery.

Paul R. Kipp, RN

Paul said, *"I'm not in this career for the gratitude but it sure feels good when it happens and you can change someone's life for the better."*

A Blessing From God

Many years ago I was working as a critical care nurse when my child's school nurse approached me. She stated bluntly and boldly, "I am retiring after 19 years and you would be great for this position." My first thought was, "Do you know what I do?"

A few months later I was opening and closing the school clinic. It was a bit challenging dealing with the many new school issues and the insulin dependent students. Daily, my heart was filled with compassion and I was always inspired with positive thoughts. A new found passion for my nursing career was discovered!

Eleven months later I was diagnosed with insulin dependent diabetes. Can you imagine the surprise on my face? I received this message as a blessing from God. My spirit as a school nurse for the last ten years has been joyful and especially so with newly diagnosed diabetic students. Each year brings a new insulin dependent diabetic student with open eyes and arms wide open! Yes, I can help you. Thank you God for giving me something so sweet!

Tammy Green, RN, BSN
Atlanta, Georgia

"Sometimes our fate resembles a fruit tree in the winter. Who would think that those branches would turn green again and blossom, but we hope it."
~ Johann Wolfgang Von Goethe

The Secret In Sally's Eyes

Getting to know Sally so early in my nursing career was truly a case of beginner's luck. I've thought of this patient – and the lessons she taught me – many times during the decades since I was fortunate enough to know her.

I met Sally on the first day of my nursing job at a state hospital. A victim of cerebral palsy, she sat slumped over in a chair near the nurses station. The chair was positioned so she could watch the nurses perform their morning duties. And watch them she did! Her eyes darted back and forth, taking in every movement. Intrigued by her bright eyes and smile, I walked over and introduced myself.

Sally, 21, had a slender, pretty face, with fair skin that drew attention to her large, dark eyes. Unfortunately, she could not control her arm or leg movements – or speak. According to her history, her communication problems were partially linked to mental retardation. I soon learned that she had been hospitalized after her mother died a few months earlier. Unable to give her the constant care she needed, her father was broken-hearted that he had to place his "little girl" in our state hospital.

Sally had two teenage brothers, Mike and Robbie, who adored her. They visited often, telling her how pretty she looked and how proud they were of her. When her dad's work schedule allowed, he'd take Sally home on the weekends. I frequently spoke with him about Sally. He told me that her physical problems worsened when she was 8-years old. When she turned 14 she could no longer speak or walk and was confined to a wheelchair. She had to leave school then.

As I cared for Sally, I grew more and more captivated by her eyes. One day I found out why......

Sally had to take her time eating and I would talk to her as I fed her. I noticed that she often looked upward as if to agree with something

135

I had said. One evening during dinner I teased her, "Is your name Lucy? No, that can't be it. Is it Janet?" I continued with names, and she looked down each time until I mentioned the name Sally. Then she looked up.

On impulse, I asked her to look up for "yes" and down for "no." I asked, "Do you like your dinner today?" She looked up. "Are you going to eat all of your carrots?" This time she looked down and smiled. I knew carrots weren't her favorite food. Her responses fueled my enthusiasm. I asked her another question, then another. Sally answered each appropriately with her eyes.

Moving her tray aside, I picked up the newspaper. I had planned to read her an article I thought she would enjoy, but then I got an idea. I asked, "Sally, can you read?" I assumed she would look down. Instead, Sally's eyes darted up, and she became so excited that she let out a shrill laugh. I held the newspaper in front of her and waited as she read. I then quizzed her about the article. Again, every answer was correct. I couldn't believe my discovery!

The entire staff shared my surprise – and my enthusiasm. Each day that week we brought in more reading materials and spent time talking with Sally. One staff member built a special book stand for Sally that could be placed in front of her chair so she could read without our help. When she needed a page turned, she would utter her characteristic shrill sound. We would kid her with comments like, "Gee Sally, you sure keep us busy now – we love you even if you are a speed reader." She would get so tickled and giggle.

When we told Sally's father our good news, he stared in disbelief. He asked her, "Would you like to come home with me today?" Her eyes darted up. And his eyes filled with tears. He told us he had known in his heart Sally understood everything he had said to her but he never dreamed she could communicate with him. "I only wish Sally's mother was here", he said quietly.

Sally and I remained close friends and several years later when I became engaged to be married. I invited Sally to my wedding. I wasn't sure she would be able to make the trip. Just before the ceremony was to begin, I peeked into the church. No sign of Sally. But as I started down the aisle, her unmistakable shrill cry filled the church. My day was complete!

I've never forgotten those eyes – or Sally. She helped me discover that my most valuable nursing tools are time and patience. Without them, it's all too easy to overlook a patient's potential – and to miss the special person within.

Peggy Humphus, LPN
Peggy is employed at Good Samaritan Society in
Las Cruces, New Mexico

Peggy said, *"I've been in nursing 38 years. Still loving it! One drop of inspiration a day will eventually fill the bucket."*

I Thought Of You Today

We were flying through storms and choppy weather - destination Seattle. The mission was to pick up a fifteen year-old girl with astrocytoma; a deadly form of incurable cancer that had spread like wildfire throughout this little girl's body. Less than two days to live: mission impossible.

I first met Lexy at her bedside and while her childlike features were delicate and soft, her feisty spirit roared like a lion that had just been prodded. This gave me hope that we would successfully accomplish our mission. The mission was to get Lexy to Las Vegas to pass away amongst friends, loved ones, and most importantly family.

Her parents were traveling with us, not an unusual occurrence, but an odd scenario none the less. They were divorced but civil for the sake of their dying daughter. Dad had been the sole care giver of this little angel for the last year. Mom had little to do with her and the effects of this horrific illness. Regardless of the circumstances when Lexy was scared she would call out for "Mommy". She snuggled her mother's cold, bony hand - drinking in her scent like a fresh picked flower. Interesting I thought. The mother who hadn't been around to wipe her child's brow, change her child's diaper, or tend to her child's needs is the person Lexy wanted in her time of need. As I looked over at dad's face, I see the hurt that he tried to hide behind tired, sleepy eyes.

As we flew through the night Lexy awoke several times crying in pain; each time asking for "Daddy". Fighting sheer exhaustion he rose and came to offer his baby daughter affection. Mommy slept through the turbulence and cries, never stirring once. It was daddy who took the seat next to his angel to soothe and comfort her. The calm before the storm was all I could think through tear stained eyes.

I thought about you today. How much our children mean to us and how the mere mention of their names produce beautiful megawatt smiles. How boastful we are of their smallest endeavors and how proud we are of their monumental achievements. I thought about you today and thought how tragic it is to watch someone you have nurtured and loves slip through you fingers like fine sand on a sunny beach. Knowing that at a moment's notice they can be quickly snatched from you. Snatched with nothing left but memories of each milestone, no matter how big or how insignificant, they were memories you were able to share. Celluloid images burned into your brain never to be erased. I thought about you today – one last time before I drifted off to sleep. My heart hurts for Lexy and I wanted to run to the ends of the earth to tell those who are important to me to live every day like it is your last. I want to hold them close, hug them, squeeze them, kiss them, but most of all tell them how much they mean to me and how much I love them; just in case one of us slips away.

Becky Pusateri, RN, MSN
Sugar Grove, Illinois

"It is well to give when asked, but it is better to give unasked, through understanding."
  ~ Kahlil Gibran - *The Prophet*

Mike

When I was an LPN I took care of an American Indian patient; Mike. He was the same age as me – 23 years old. He had been doing drugs and went into respiratory arrest. Apparently when he was found he was resuscitated, but had already suffered anoxic brain damage. Consequently he was paralyzed, unable to speak, talk, or do anything for himself. By the time I was assigned as his primary care nurse he already had a g-tube, Foley, and was losing weight and muscle mass. He had problems maintaining his temperature. Either it would be too high and he required frequent bed baths, or it would be too low and we had to provide him a warming blanket.

One of the other nurses refused to care for him, "Because he did it to himself and he deserved to be like that." So each day I was on shift I was assigned to Mike. During the three months I cared for him in the hospital, I recruited three nurses' aides to help me ensure Mike was turned, fed, and kept clean. One of us was almost always on shift, so we knew that he was being cared for. Sadly, the unfortunate nurse with the hateful attitude was not the only one who felt that way. We developed a system to know if his g-tube care had been done. It required frequent drain sponge dressing changes due to leakage, and we placed two levels of dressing with a star (for nights) and a sun (for days) on the bottom level.

During the time I cared for him I found out he could see and hear, and he began to follow me with his eyes. I talked to him about anything and everything while doing daily bedside care. I discovered Mike liked rock music and we would put the radio onto the rock station. Some of the nurses put it on country, and he would turn his head to the wall and clench his eyes shut.

Basically, he was "locked in", able to feel, hear, and see, but unable to communicate or move. I figured since humans only use 10 to 15% of their brains, and he had burned out probably 10 to 15% of his, that there was still a good 80% left to use to relearn how to talk and move. I told him and the nurse aides this and we began a crusade to get him back to being able to do things for himself.

We started doing range of motion exercises and working with him, getting him up into a chair and taking him out of the room and letting him get some sunshine. I got him to communicate with eye blinks: one being "no" and two being "yes". He was subsequently able to answer questions and let us know what he needed. He would clench his eyes really hard so we would not miss what his answer was to our questions. After a time he was able to squeeze two fingers of his right hand when doing the neurological checks. When this happened we all were so excited and happy!

The aides told me when I was off he would watch the door each morning to see if I was coming in. I let him know when I was going to be off and when I was coming back. Once I asked him if all the drugs were worth it, and he turned his head away and would not look at me or interact for the rest of the day.

When he first came in he had really long hair that we would wash and put in a braid for him. Somewhere along the way, his Aunt came in and cut his braid off. According to the aide on duty at the time the Aunt told him, "You don't deserve this braid. You have disgraced our tribe." I was off when this happened and Teresa, one of my faithful aides, told me Mike cried for an hour after his Aunt left. He apparently would not open his eyes and kept his face turned away the rest of the day.

During his stay there were funding issues and no rehabilitation facility could be found to take him. One day, after being off work for three days, I went to Mike's room and found it empty. I immediately went to the nurses' station to get report and find out where he went. Mike's physician was standing there, saw me, and said, "Oh good. Here you are, come with me. I have something to tell you." I thought, "Oh no, Mike has gotten worse and had to leave for Tulsa." The doctor took me to the cafeteria, got me a cup of coffee, and sat down with me. All I could think was, "Man, this has to be bad for *this* doctor to be getting *me* coffee." Then he said, "I have seen the kind of care you have been giving Mike and I want you to know that I really appreciate it." He continued by saying, "I want to tell you what happened two days ago. Mike's Aunt came in and told him 'our tribe is out of money and so are two others that we have borrowed money from for your care. You are never going to get better, so it is ok with us if you just go ahead and die.' She left and he then died within 20 minutes."

I just sat there in shock and said, "Can the human will be so strong to just die like that?" The doctor said, "Apparently so" patted me on the back, thanked me again, and left. I was unable to attend the funeral, as it was in a town about 120 miles away and I had to work. I did send a card to his family signed, "The nurse with the long hair", which is what all of the Indian patients called me.

Sandra Grant, RN, MSN, FNP-C
Lubbock, Texas

"Do the best you can in every task, no matter how unimportant it may seem at the time. No one learns more about a problem than the person at the bottom."

~ Sandra Day O'Connor

6

Philosophies To Keep With You

"What great thing would you attempt if you knew you could not fail?"

~ Robert H. Schuller

"The greatest discovery of my generation is that a human being can alter his life by altering his attitude."
  ~ William James

"A man cannot be comfortable without his own approval."
  ~ Mark Twain

"From what we get, we can make a living; what we give, however, makes a life."
  ~ Arthur Ashe – *Days of Grace*

"You can't build a reputation on what you are going to do."
  ~ Henry Ford

"On this earth, in the final analysis, each of us gets exactly what he deserves. But only the successful recognize this."
  ~ Georges Simenon

"I like the dreams of the future better than the history of the past."
  ~ Thomas Jefferson

"Yesterday is experience. Tomorrow is hope. Today is getting from one to the other as best we can."
  ~ John M. Henry

Printed in the United States
207612BV00001B/120/P